Coconut
Cracked Open

CHRISTINE SCHANG

Coconut
Cracked Open

FOOD • HEALTH • DIET • BEAUTY
THE NEW REVOLUTION IN FEELING GOOD AND LOOKING GREAT

NEW
HOLLAND

CHRISTINE SCHANG

Contents

Introduction

From an early age, about the time when I began to see the world around me outside myself, I always questioned how our body worked and found basic biology and food technology of the time not adequate to satisfy my inquisitive mind.

Initially I studied health, moving into nursing, and during this time I came to the personal conclusion that I was only patching up those who were already experiencing illness and disease, not preventing it. So I went on to pursue clinical massage and other ways to reduce stress and pain. And this in turn inspired a journey towards learning how and what to do to prevent or delay the onset of illness and disease.

Recognising that you cannot promise to totally prevent disease and illness, I still needed to feel that I could educate and make a positive contribution in preventative medicine.

My true driving force to learn and study naturopathy came through my children and my father. I felt strongly compelled, as parents often do, to offer them the healthiest path for their life journey, and launched into study for five years to obtain my Bachelor of Health Science.

We all know that our journey never truly ends in the quest for a healthy lifestyle, and so I continue to challenge myself and expand my knowledge with continued professional education in areas such as homeopathy, Bowen technique and Dorn therapy. The journey continues with this book on coconuts, one of Mother Nature's wonder products.

The coconut:
a short history

Botanically, the coconut is actually a fruit (drupe) not a true nut. COCONUT (*Cocos nucifera*) is of the family Arecaceae (the palm family). The spelling cocoanut is an archaic form of the word 'cocos'. The term 'cocos' is derived from both the Portuguese and Spanish *cocos*, which referred to a mythological bogeyman or ghost with a pumpkin head that would hide in the shadows, watching out for mischievous children. It was associated with fear and a way for parents to manage naughty children. They would hollow out pumpkins, cut eyes and grinning mouths and put lights into them and leave them in dark places to frighten people. When the Portuguese and Spanish sailors saw these brown shrivelled head-like fruit with what looks like two eyes and a mouth (a grinning face) with coarse patchy hair and the likeness to their myth they called them *Cocos*. Samuel Johnson's *Dictionary of the English Language* spelled the fruit cocoanut. When chocolate was introduced into England, many people thought Johnson had confused the nuts with the cacao beans, later called cocoa.

The 'grinning face', from the three small holes on the coconut shell, which resemble two eyes and a nose, are actually the tree germination pores (stoma) that are the trademark of the coconut. The coconut has three layers. The exocarp (outer) and mesocarp (middle) make up the 'husk' of the coconut plus the endocarp (centre). Coconuts sold in the shops of many countries often have the exocarp (outermost layer) removed. The mesocarp is composed of a strong coarse fibre, called coir, which has many traditional and commercial uses, such as rope. Even now, the coconut husks, as an end product, can be shredded and used as garden products. The endocarp is a shell that has three germination pores (stoma) or 'eyes' that are clearly visible on its outside surface once the husk is removed. Inside, this endocarp is where the meat and the juice are protected.

Grown in as many as 90 countries, the coconut palm grows up to 90 feet high, in the tall genus species. There are two natural sub-groups in the species, simpy referred to as 'Tall' and 'Dwarf'. Each producing region has its own selection, e.g. 'Indian Tall' or Jamaican Tall'. The tall cultivars are grown commercially because they live longer and are higher yielding than the dwarf cultivars. The coconut palm thrives on sandy soils, preferring areas with abundant sunlight and regular rainfall (59–98½in/150–250cm annually). Coconuts also need high humidity (70–80% or above) and a mean annual temperature of 81°F (27°C), for the best possible production growth and do well in areas with an average summer temperature between 82 and 99°F (28 and 37°C). A healthy full-sized coconut weighs about 3.2lb (1.44kg)—no surprise then that a coconut falling on the head of an unsuspecting person can be fatal.

Coconut fruit in the wild are light, buoyant and highly water resistant, and have migrated significant distances. The oldest fossils known of the modern coconut date from the Eocene period from around 37 to 55 million years ago and were found in Australia and India. However, older palm fossils called Nipa fruit have been found in the Americas. The Philippines and Indonesia are the largest producers of coconuts, followed by India. The coconut still has natural pests that can threaten its production, from butterflies, weevils and beetles, mite infestations that could wipe out 90 per cent of production crops if not managed carefully.

Given that the coconut has been around for such a long time it's not surprising that it is not only used as a food substance, but has been adapted for use in moisturisers, emulsions in cream bases and its anti-bacterial, anti-fungal and anti-viral properties have been discovered.

It is classified as a 'functional food' because it provides many health benefits beyond its nutritional content. The coconut palm is highly valued in Asia and the Pacific Islands, where coconut oil is considered to be the cure for all illness. Used as both a source of food and medicine, the coconut tree is referred to as the 'Tree of Life'.

Coconut:
Its healing properties

The coconut is known for its versatility as seen in the many domestic, commercial and industrial uses of its different parts.

Processing of coconut

Over the years, various methods of extraction have been developed to obtain the oil from coconut. How the oil is extracted can affect the quality of the oil and how it is used. The initial process is to remove the meat from the shell and then to separate the oil from the meat by one of two methods: dry or wet extraction. The age of the harvested coconut can significantly affect the quality and yield of the oil produced. The variation of age to harvest is between two and 20 months of growth. After extraction, oil then may undergo various treatments to extend the shelf life of the oil and further separate the oil, using only properties that they need, in combination with other chemicals, to make another product. Some of these oil extractions are suitable only for industry use while other treatments to the oil allow the oil to be used for consumption in food and for health benefits at home. Following is a brief description of the extraction, processing and refinements that coconut oil can undergo to be used commercially.

Dry process

Dry processing requires the meat to be extracted from the shell and dried using fire, sunlight or kilns to create copra. This copra is now the raw material to extract the oil from.

Copra is pressed to extract the oil initially and then the remaining pulp may be further dissolved using solvents such as Hexane, a liquid petroleum product. This second process is used to increase the yield from the remaining copra that milling can't remove to produce the coconut oil .

Wet process

The wet process uses raw coconut meat rather than dried copra. The protein in the coconut creates an emulsion of oil and water. The difficulty is breaking up the emulsion to recover the oil. This used to be done by boiling the emulsion for a prolonged period, producing a discoloured oil, which was not economical. Today pre-treatments such as heat, cold, acid, salts, enzymes, pressure and shock waves break up the emulsion, then centrifuges are used to spin off the oil from the water, which is then discarded.

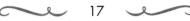

Refined, bleached and deodorised (RBD)

This 'crude' coconut oil resulting from wet or dry processing is not suitable for consumption because it contains contaminants and is processed to refine, bleach and deodorise with further heating and filtering. The refined coconut oil has no coconut taste or aroma and the oil is used for cooking, commercial food processing, cosmetic, industrial and pharmaceutical purposes. One of the refinement processes of coconut oil is to increase its melting point. Since virgin and RBD coconut oils melt at 75°F (24°C) with a smoking point of 350°F (177°C). Foods containing coconut oil tend to melt in warm climates. A higher melting point is desirable in these warm climates, so the oil is hydrogenated. The melting point of hydrogenated coconut oil is 97–104°F (36–40°C) with a smoking point of 450°F (232°C). In the process of hydrogenation, unsaturated fats (monounsaturated and polyunsaturated fatty acids) are combined with hydrogen in a catalytic process to make them more saturated. With this process, the oil is transformed into trans-fatty acids—these are the bad fats that we avoid for our health because of the way our body processes the oil. Hydrogenated coconut oil is used commercially in salty snacks, biscuits, baked goods, cereals, cakes and pastries, to name a few, as it is cheaper to produce than virgin coconut oil and increases the shelf life of products and reduces the need for refrigeration

Fractionation

Fractionation is what chemical manufacturers do to extract a portion of a natural molecule or chemical. Fractionated coconut oil is a fraction of the whole oil, in which the different medium-chain fatty acids are separated for specific uses. Lauric acid, found naturally in coconut oil, is often removed because of its anti-bacterial, anti-viral and anti-fungal properties and is valuable for industrial and medical purposes. The fractionation of coconut oil may also be used to make caprylic/capric triglyceride oil. This triglyceride oil, like lauric acid, is frequently used for medical applications, special diets and cosmetics, and is sometimes also used as a carrier oil for fragrances.

Natural coconut oil and water

Coconut oil and water possess healing properties and both have been extensively used in traditional medicine among Asian and Pacific populations, long before science discovered its commercial uses. Our body processes food we ingest in very specific ways, breaking down molecules, transporting, using and eventually eliminating the portions our body can't use. By using coconut water and oil in their natural state, we are using a healthy nutritional product that our body benefits from. When we interfere with that process to extend the life of a product by changing its chemical structure, it interferes with the way our body chemistry identifies with the product and how it then metabolises and processes the chemical structure and nutritional aspect of a product.

An example of this is in the hydrogenation of coconut oil that changes a medium-chained saturated fat that our body can metabolise and use efficiently into trans fatty acids that we now know contributes to many health conditions because of the way our body has to metabolise this altered product.

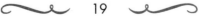

Coconut water

If you've ever been on a holiday to a tropical paradise, then you would have seen the wonderful coconut palm laden with its bounty of luscious fruit, the coconut. And chances are you have tried this feast of nature, a refreshing treat. Coconut water is a versatile product that can be used in cooking, such as soups, desserts and main dishes, and is wonderful in juices and drinks to help boost your health and dietary regime. Incorporated into your fitness and exercise program it acts naturally as a great recovery tool and hydration fluid.

To get to the coconut water, a hole is bored into the coconut to provide access to the liquid and it is either poured into a glass or drunk straight from the fruit itself. The liquid is thicker than water and very sweet. Coconut water is composed of many naturally occurring bioactive enzymes. These enzymes help with your digestion and metabolism.

Coconuts are different from any other fruits because they contain a large quantity of liquid. In general, young and slightly immature coconuts, known as tender-nuts or jelly-nuts, are harvested at about five to seven months for drinking. The water is obtained by opening a tender, green, healthy and undamaged coconut. Inside, its clear liquid is sweet, sterile and composed of unique chemicals such as sugars, vitamins, minerals in trace amounts, electrolytes such as sodium and potassium, enzymes, amino acids, cytokine, and phyto-hormones again in trace amounts.

Coconut water contains a very good amount of electrolytes, sodium, potassium and a small amount of vitamin C, which is a water-soluble antioxidant. These are the marketed health aspects of coconut water that have given the liquid its popularity.

Coconut water can be purchased in cans, plastic or glass bottles, sometimes with coconut pulp or coconut jelly included. Bottled coconut water has a shelf life of 24 months, so commercial coconut water could be enhanced with additives to ensure the product has a good shelf life. Fresh is, as always, the best assurance of quality as coconut water does perish and break down just as it's supposed to do. You can obtain fresh green coconuts from your supermarket that are ready to take home and use as you need.

Coconut water is also widely advertised as isotonic water, or an electrolyte replacement by the health and fitness industry. It is the naturally occurring electrolytes in just the right combination that make this product just perfect as a training supplement, in addition to regular water.

But what does isotonic actually mean? Here's just a little chemistry to explain. Most intravenous therapy solutions that are used in hospitals and medical centres are isotonic. Isotonic solutions are designed to match the make-up of your intracellular fluid and are equal in osmotic pressure inside and outside your cells. This prevents any fluid shifting in and out of your cells, reducing and preventing dehydration. So, in a nutshell, coconut water is naturally similar to the composition of your blood and it mixes easily with blood. This is possible because the coconut water has a balance of sugar and electrolytes that makes it possible to be used in the bloodstream efficiently and effectively.

For hundreds of years, defence and medical forces have used and still use coconut water as a plasma replacement and hydration medium when extreme circumstances require it in the field. Coconut water can even be injected straight into the veins (but don't try this at home). The cavity inside a coconut, where the coconut water is found, is sterile until opened. During the Pacific campaign in World War II, coconut water was used as a substitute for saline drips when they ran out of supplies and served as an emergency short-term intravenous hydration fluid. A needle was inserted into a young coconut and dripped directly into the vein.

So how can you use it at home? You can cook with it and drink it, incorporating it into your healthy dietary routine. It is safe to use every day in moderation or when on a controlled diet, in your quest to either lose weight or to give yourself an energy boost.

If you are using it for weight loss, remember that this product still contains calories from the carbohydrate content: 1 cup contains approximately 50 calories. So be wary and stick primarily to your clean, filtered, fresh 2–4½ pints (1–2 litres) of water and just add coconut water as part of this intake to make your routine more interesting, tasty and give you an energy boost.

If you follow the contemporary paleolithic diet, then you could enjoy this fundamental product for health juices. You could enjoy one per day, perhaps two if you are incorporating it into a fitness regime. For example, you could have some coconut water on most days to kickstart your day, and then treat and activate your liver with my Invigorating Juice (see recipe) or, on the days that you're working out, you could include the Energiser Chaser (see recipe) within 30 minutes of your workout to support and replenish your energy levels and support tissue healing. It is amazing how one juice will process through your body, helping so many organs to do their job.

Coconut water is also an excellent hydration product, but should be incorporated into a generally well-balanced, healthy eating plan. Everything in life should be in moderation and our bodies appreciate balance throughout our lives. This product can provide nutrition to assist that balance so long as it's not overused or abused. Like anything new, exciting and good for us we don't want to use so much of it that we lose the benefits it is offering.

Also, please be warned: if you are a person taking medication, have a history of heart disease and kidney disease and are on a restricted potassium intake or just need to be cautious of your potassium intake, then this will not be a product for you, no matter how natural. So be wise and sensible with your health and your body's specific needs.

Coconut water's anti-bacterial properties, lauric acid, can be helpful with symptoms of mild urinary tract infections but, if this is a recurring problem, please be advised to look further into the source of the problem by seeing your general health practitioner, to determine the true cause and take long-term preventative steps.

Coconut oil

Natural health practitioners have long understood the health benefits associated with virgin/raw, organic, cold-pressed coconut oil and now it seems the secret is out about coconut oil and its amazing benefits.

Coconut oil is solid at room temperature (65°F/18°C) and is a clean, white, silky smooth oil with a delightfully aromatic natural fragrance. When it is gently warmed (about 75°F/24°C) it forms a crystal-clear liquid that is luscious and creamy in sensation.

To understand coconut oil a little better, I am going to share with you why you are making a healthy decision to use this oil if you choose to.

Fats and oils are composed of molecules called fatty acids, which are

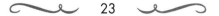

made of long chains of carbon atoms with hydrogen atoms attached; three fatty acids joined together form a triglyceride molecule. Some fatty acids are smaller than others. These fatty acids are classified as short-chain fatty acids (SCFA), medium-chain fatty acids (MCFA) and long-chain fatty acids (LCFA).

Most of the fats and oils in our diet are composed of LCFA, whether they're unsaturated or saturated. The size of these molecules is very important because our bodies process and metabolise each fat differently depending on its size.

The important difference between the digestion MCFAs and the LCFAs is that the LCFAs need digestive enzymes (pancreatic acids) to break them down into smaller lipoproteins before they can pass through the intestinal walls and be released into the bloodstream. These LCFAs spend more time in the body waiting to be broken down by available pancreatic enzymes and then used by the body as fuel. If your body has other sources of fuel for the liver and energy while waiting to convert these LCFAs they can be stored as fat or attracted to plaque in your arteries from inflammation, adding to the build-up of arterial plaque.

Saturated fats found in coconut oil are used in the body as an important source of energy and an integral part of the cell membrane structure. Short- to medium-chain fatty acids are more water-soluble than long-chain fatty acids and thus require less energy for the body to absorb and use. They are freely absorbed into the bloodstream without the need for pancreatic enzymes and so are a quick source of energy, raising the metabolism of the body. These SCFAs reduce your metabolic load that allows the liver to optimise its detoxifying functions, bile production and regulation of blood sugar levels.

Lauric acid

Lauric acid is an MCFA found in coconut oil that protects the fruit, similar to that of a natural pesticide. When we ingest this oil, our bodies convert lauric acid to monolaurin. Monolaurin works by disrupting the lipid membranes in organisms like fungus, bacteria and viruses, which in turn, kills them. In our body, that forms natural anti-bacterial and anti-fungal properties, which means that these fats have the ability to be anti-viral, anti-fungal and anti-bacterial both internally and externally.

MCFAs

There are only a few dietary sources of medium-chain fatty acids, the primary source being tropical oils, particularly palm kernel and coconut oils. That is why coconut oil is different from other oils and this is the secret to many of its healing properties.

Coconut oil has medium- and short-chain fatty acids that are digested and absorbed differently to long-chain fatty acids and are a healthier fatty acid.

Cold-pressed is best

Cold-pressed virgin coconut oil has that dreamy, creamy aroma. Virgin coconut oil (VCO) can be produced from fresh coconut meat, milk or residue. To produce cold-pressed oil the fresh coconut 'meat' is removed from the shell and washed. It then goes through a process of either wet-milling or drying the residue and a screw press extracts the oil.

The lower temperature of extraction in the pressing of the coconut oil and the minimal processing of the oil mean that the coconut oil can retain its important antioxidant properties. Antioxidants slow down free radical formations in the body that are made from food and chemicals we metabolise that can damage our cell membranes.

In searching for a quality product that uses cold-pressed extraction, check out the common coconut oil products and their websites and read how the oil is processed. The quality products will usually have very proud producers who are more than happy to explain how their product is made.

VCO is completely non-toxic and can be used as an oil for frying, as it has a very high smoke point and the smoking point for clean virgin coconut oil is usually 350°F (177°C).

Virgin coconut oil is one of the few oils that is not damaged when heated to temperatures used in cooking, frying and baking. In our constant demand to use products commercially, coconut oil in its refined state can attain a smoking point of 459°F (232°C). For our domestic use, the lower temperature is better for our health. I hope we don't need to cook our food at smoking point to achieve nutritious food at home.

This lovely oil can be blended easily into smoothies, dips and also used in many raw food recipes. I have included a few in this book.

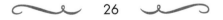

Reducing your toxic load

Most of us are walking chemical factories. Everything from the food we eat and digest, to the water and fluid we drink, to the air we breathe can contain some element of chemicals that may cause an imbalance to our health and wellbeing.

Our skin is the largest eliminatory organ in the body and is a two-way membrane. Toxins are eliminated through the skin via perspiration and absorbed through the skin, into the body's systemic circulation, through hair follicles and sebaceous glands (not through sweat glands). You may try to eat healthy foods and drink clean, filtered water but what about the other products you effectively consume, such as personal care products and cosmetics.

Cosmetic manufacturers are not supposed to claim that their products penetrate our skin (even though we all know these products can be absorbed that way). If they did, then lots of chemical compounds in products that we use every day would have to be labelled a 'drug' and be governed by much stricter regulations. Manufacturers get around this by using products that come from natural sources, such as lauric acid from coconut. By changing or by adding something to its chemical structure in a laboratory, such as attaching a sulphate bond to the lauric acid from coconut, the original good product, in this case lauric acid, is now able to be used in a chemically processed form as a detergent and foaming agent found in shampoo, toothpaste, body wash, soaps and moisturisers. Yet it has the potential to cause skin irritation in sensitive individuals. Who doesn't like a foaming body wash and shampoo—it makes us feel like we are cleaner when products foam and lather up. Yet the very thing that makes us feel 'clean' is doing us more harm than good.

Most of our commercial personal care products boast about being organic or low allergenic. Always read the labels; however, you may need a good magnifying glass for this as the print size and number of ingredients on small bottles is not always easily read with the naked eye. Make use of the web to find out about any of the ingredients in your personal care products, to see what side effects they may have, such as skin irritation.

These personal care products might also contain ingredients in seemingly harmless quantities yet cumulatively they add to our toxic load and may account for unexplained irritation or other seemingly unrelated symptoms that are difficult to pinpoint because it could be the combinations of products and their chemical reactions that is the actual cause.

Think, just for a moment, about what you are wearing other than your clothes as you head out into the world every morning.

• You wake up and brush your teeth, using mouthwash and toothpaste that contain detergent additives, flavours, alcohol and colours.
• you have a shower—using shower gel/body wash and shampoo and

conditioner—products that could contain sodium lauryl sulfate.

- you style and dry your hair, using hair gel straightening balm, styling mousse and hairspray perhaps.
- have you cleaned your face? Look at the long list on those bottles.
- then you might apply some make-up: foundation, mascara, eye shadow, blush, lipstick. Lovely chemical concoctions that are likely to have petrochemical additives, colours and perfumes to make them all smell fragrant and attractive.
- don't forget the deodorant, anti-perspirant and perfume
- now it's time to get dressed and what did you wash your clothes in? Detergent?
- Did you use fabric softener? Strong detergents to remove oil and dirt and lots of synthetic fragrances to make them smell nice.
- off to breakfast: packaged juice, cereals, processed, enhanced milk of some kind with low fat, no fat, added vitamins and flavours and natural colours.
- then off to the car to sit and absorb all those exogenous oestrogens that are released from the plastic and synthetics inside cars and released by heat and trapped until you open the door.

This is just before work. What about the rest of the day! Do you wonder why you might feel unwell? You're doing this day in, day out, year after year after year, and marketing is targeting the younger generations all the time. What age were you when you used your first deodorant, and how old were your parents? Ask them and you may find it was at an older age.

What is your load limit? Why, after years of being fine and not really changing anything in your diet or routine, are you developing symptoms that are silently creeping up on you?

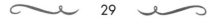

Symptoms such as:

- waking tired after what seems like a full night's sleep, again and again.
- suffering allergic symptoms earlier than usual or longer or more severely, or even developing allergic symptoms you've never suffered from before, such as sinusitis, seasonal rhinitis or hay fever?
- reacting to skin products and changing brands until you find one that isn't as irritating? Do you tell yourself that the product doesn't suit your skin, or is perhaps the interaction of chemicals in combined products you are using?

If you want to make some changes to the products you buy there are websites that list product alternatives.

Emollients

Emollients serve two functions: they prevent dryness and protect the skin, acting as a barrier and healing agent. Water is the best emollient, but because it evaporates quickly it is ineffective. It needs to be held on the skin by emollient oils in what is called an emulsion. Natural emollients actually nourish the skin. They are metabolised by the skin's own enzymes and absorbed into it. They are readily biodegradable and are of edible quality. Coconut oil is one kind of natural emollient.

Coconuts are used in the beauty industry in moisturisers and body butters because coconut oil, due to its chemical structure, is readily absorbed by the skin. The coconut shell may also be ground down and added to products for exfoliation of dead skin.

Why not consider swapping some of the complicated products you use on your skin for the simple and inexpensive alternatives that coconut oil can provide?

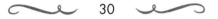

Coconut can help

Beauty products made with coconut oil

Homemade Deodorant

¼ cup baking soda (will act as a deodoriser)

¼ cup arrowroot powder or cornflour starch (will act as an antiperspirant)

10–15 drops essential oil of your choice

2 tablespoons coconut oil (will act as an anti-bacterial and deodoriser)

- Mix baking soda and arrowroot together.
- Add the essentail oil and coconut oil gradually, mixing well, until you make a paste.
- Pour into a clean jar.
- Use an ice-block stick or your fingers to get the deodorant out of the container. There are no rules, just make sure you use enough under your arms to keep you dry all day long.

Eye-makeup remover: Warm up a small amount of coconut oil, apply to a cotton eye pad and gently wipe away your make-up.

Night cream: Use coconut oil as a night cream to moisturise after cleansing. You won't need very much as the oil melts with the warmth of your fingers and leaves your skin soft.

Lip balm: Rub some coconut oil on your lips as a natural lip balm.

Facial scrub: Mix desiccated coconut and coconut oil together to form a paste. Massage over your face as you would any scrub and wash off in the shower. This can be used as a body scrub as well.

Body scrub: Add ½ cup of sea salt and a few drops of your favourite 100 per cent pure essential oil. Gradually add some raw organic coconut oil until you have a paste consistency and you have a natural body scrub that will exfoliate and moisturise at the same time. Whip in some shea butter for a soothing body balm after your body exfoliation.

Hair conditioner: Coconut oil is an effective and inexpensive deep-conditioning treatment for hair. It will combat frizz, moisturise dry hair and add shine and strength to your locks. Best of all, it contains no chemicals or alcohol. It's a cost-effective product and reduces your toxic load.

When your hair needs a wash, just before bed, rub coconut oil into your scalp and hair, or just your hair if you prefer. Leave in overnight and shampoo as usual in the morning.

Deeper conditioning treatment: Gently shampoo your hair and rinse it with warm water. Squeeze excess water from hair with a towel. Apply a generous amount of coconut oil to damp hair. Massage the oil into your scalp and then distribute oil down to the tips. If you have long hair, use a bit more coconut oil. You can use a wide-toothed comb to distribute the oil through your hair.

Cover your hair with either a plastic shower cap or wrap your head in plastic wrap and cover in a towel to keep warm. This will ensure that the oil penetrates your hair.

Leave in for 30–60 minutes, giving you enough time to clean the house! Wash hair with a gentle shampoo, condition and dry as usual. Treat your hair to this deep condition every few weeks.

Other uses for coconut oil: Topically, coconut oil can help skin heal faster after injury or infection. After the initial heat is gone it can also help speed the healing of sunburn.

Rub some onto your hands after doing the dishes to avoid dry skin and as a general moisturiser, it can help your nails to grow strong and long. Mixed with tea tree, eucalyptus, catnip, rosemary or mint essential oils it can be used as a natural bug repellent.

As a safe nappy rash cream: just rub some on baby's bottom—or to treat cradle cap. Apply small amounts over the scaly scalp at night and massage gently to allow the oil to be absorbed. Then wash off in the morning bath. Repeat this process until the scalp is lovely and clean.

Coconut oil has been found to lighten age spots when rubbed directly on the skin over time. Coconut oil as a moisturiser may also assist in the prevention of stretch marks during pregnancy.

Dry cracked heels, rough elbows and knees: Mix some coconut oil with salt and scrub your feet, elbows or knees to remove dry skin. Wash off in the shower and moisturise with a small amount of oil before bed. Remember that dry skin can come from an essential fatty acid deficiency, so taking the oil internally daily can lubricate your skin inside and out and you may find you don't suffer from the same dry skin as you did before.

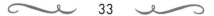

The Importance of Dental Hygiene

Our oral hygiene is a very important aspect of our health. We brush our teeth usually twice a day for most of our lives for that clean fresh breath and healthy white teeth and gums. A part of reducing your toxic load can be as simple as exchanging your commercial toothpaste for a homemade version with coconut oil. Coconut oil contains natural lauric acid, a fatty acid with anti-bacterial properties essential for good oral hygiene.

Homemade Toothpaste with Coconut Oil

There are lots of different home recipes readily available on the web but this is just a sample to get you going. Start small and if you like the product you can double the quantity to suit. Play around with the mixture and you will come up with one that really works for your.

1–2 drops stevia liquid (optional, available in most supermarket chains)

2 tablespoons cold-pressed coconut oil (to act as the anti-bacterial agent)

2 tablespoons baking soda (to act as the abrasive agent to remove plaque build-up)

5–10 drops essential oil—peppermint, orange or lemon (make sure you only use 100% pure oils)

1 tablespoon calcium/magnesium powder (optional—usually you would take a muscle or bone supplement internally but there is no reason it can't be added here)

- Mix all ingredients together in a bowl. Blend and whip until smooth and creamy. You can mix smaller quantities by hand, but you might find a hand blender useful for larger amounts.
- Pour into a jar and seal it up until ready to use. Glass is best but you can get great plastic jars at the craft store that hold just the right amount. For hygiene purposes, even for just one person, try using a wooden

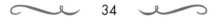

popsicle stick as an applicator from jar to the toothbrush (also available in party shops and craft stores).

Hint: After brushing, allow your toothbrush to dry, reducing bacterial growth, and get a new brush every three months.

Oil pulling using coconut oil

Oil pulling is an age-old Ayurvedic process. The theory is that the oil draws out the bacteria in the mouth and the natural lauric acid cleans out those nooks and crannies that brushes can't get to. This method of oral hygiene can lower the amount of strep mutans, the main bacteria that causes tooth decay. With regular practice you will find you have cleaner, fresher breath and whiter teeth, as well as overall better oral health (and overall health).

This process works better in the morning on an empty stomach before drinking any liquids (including water). If, for some reason, it is absolutely not possible for you to practise this method in the morning, you can do it on an empty stomach at any time of the day. An empty stomach means your food has been digested completely, ideally after three or four hours of you taking any food.

If you do this first thing in the morning, you may feel a little queasy from the oil pulling experience until you get used to it. Noticed your breath before brushing? This is because there are lots of gathered bacteria at this time.

Step 1: Warm one tablespoon of cold-pressed coconut oil and hold in your mouth.

Step 2: Swish the oil around in your mouth without swallowing it. Move it around in your mouth and through your teeth, as if it was mouthwash (don't tilt your head back to gargle though). You'll find that the oil will start to get watery as your saliva mixes with it, so keep swishing constantly. If your jaw muscles get sore while swishing, you're putting too much into it. Relax your jaw muscles and use your tongue to help move the liquid around the inside of your mouth. When you do this correctly, you'll feel very comfortable. It's ok to start doing this for just a few minutes and build up to 20 minutes. There is no right way or wrong way to swish and pull oil. Don't focus on doing it right.If you have the unbearable urge to swallow, or if it becomes too unpleasant, spit out and try again the next day. It can be a bit unpleasant at first when you're not used to it, but soon it won't be bothersome at all, just like brushing your teeth. Start with just a few minutes each time and increase as you become more comfortable with the technique.

When the oil has become saturated with the toxins it has pulled out, it may become whitish and a thinner, milky consistency. Each time you oil pull, it can take a different amount of time to get to that point, so up to 20 minutes is a general rule of thumb, but you can experiment with this. If you need to swallow a bit during oil pulling, the toxins being drawn out can usually be handled by the digestive system and eliminated properly. If you feel the urge to swallow, just spit out the whole thing and have another go the next day. Don't stress if the oil doesn't turn white straight away, the viscosity and colour should change significantly, but remember this depends on so many individual factors, and can even be slightly different each time. A milky or creamy colour is fine.

Step 3: As the end of the oil pulling session approaches, spit the oil out, then rinse the mouth with warm salt water (try to find a clean salt as salt can also have lots of contaminants in cheaper brands). Salt water rinsing isn't absolutely necessary, but is very helpful as an antimicrobial and to soothe any inflammation and has proven to be effective in rinsing out any toxins which may be left out in the mouth.

Step 4: It's important to brush after oil pulling and clean the mouth thoroughly after toxins are drawn out with salt and water as explained before.

The important thing to keep in mind when doing this or any new routine in your life to change your health is that doing this for just a few minutes each time is better than not trying at all. Doing something small even for a few minutes is going to be doing something helpful. Change is a gradual process so be kind to yourself and you will achieve change.

When you first try this method you may want to use a smaller amount and for just a few minutes at a time until you are more comfortable with the sensations and time. I try to leave it in while I am showering, or getting out my gear for the day. Try starting this method several times per week initially and build up to every second day or daily if you like. See if you notice any changes in your wellbeing in general. It's important to have two separate tooth brushes one for after oil pulling and one for regular cleaning at night because of the bacterial component.

Children can also do this with a smaller quantity of oil, provided they have control and practise not to swallow the oil, probably not under about eight-years-old perhaps.

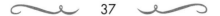

Allergic reaction to coconut products?

Unfortunately, more people than not are experiencing sensitivities or full-blown allergies to certain foods. Two most common food groups that cause allergies are dairy and nuts. People who suffer from tree nut allergies usually do fine with coconuts. If you are one of those who suffer reactions then always consider that you may react to coconut and tread cautiously. You will know better than most how to test for reactions and what the signs and symptom will be. Tree nuts and coconuts come from different species families and they produce completely different proteins. Coconut is classified as a fruit and seed rather than a nut. Botanists classify them as dry drupes. Dry drupes are fruits that have an outer fleshy layer with an encased seed in the middle.

Contact reactions are the most common and it is likely to be those fractionised products from coconut that are present in cosmetics including some shampoos, moisturisers, soaps, cleansers and hand-washing liquids. As with any contact dermatitis, a red irritation may occur soon after contact or an itchy blistering rash may arise a day or two after contact with the allergen and take several days to resolve. Regardless if you have a food allergy or a contact allergy your body is reacting to certain proteins. When you come into contact with these proteins, your immune system responds by releasing an antibody called IgE (immunoglobulin E). The proteins from the food or substance trigger the reaction. The more common symptoms include:

- internal or external itching
- tingling sensation and/or an area of swollen tissue
- sensation of feeling hot
- swollen glands

If contact dermatitis to coconut products is suspected or if you've never had coconut before and you're not sure whether or not you may have a coconut allergy, you can do a simple patch test as an appropriate method for diagnosis. Take some coconut oil or milk and rub a little on the inside of your upper arm. Massage in well. Wait a day or so and see if a reaction occurs. If all is ok then take tiny amounts internally and again wait to see if you have any reactions.

Treat our pets well

Pets can also enjoy the benefits as coconut oil is safe for your pets. They will have gorgeous, lustrous, glossy coats and healthy digestive systems. Coconut oil can also assist with worm control. Just mix either a quarter, a half or a teaspoon of oil into your pet's food daily, depending on the size of your pet. Most animals like the flavour and will lick it easily.

Worms and parasites: Children and adults can suffer from worm infestation and other parasites. Remember that if you have pets then you need to treat them as well as yourself. If you are around other people's pets check that they are regularly treated as well. Once detected, don't think anyone is excluded in the treatment. I would treat everyone for eight weeks, twice per day, internally and include other immune supporting herbs available from your local naturopath as well. Juices and smoothies with the oil and the water can be a great way to get children interested in being more compliant.

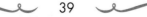

Coconut and its wonderful products

Coconut by-products

Of course, there's more to coconut than just oil and water. There are also a whole variety of coconut products available, including: coconut milk, coconut cream, coconut water, coconut flour, coconut flakes and coconut butter.

With the high demand and necessity for gluten-free products, you can use coconut oil and other coconut by-products in the pantry. I will give you a general insight into how they can benefit your health and be used in cooking and personal care products.

Coconut sugar is not the same as palm sugar

In some areas, predominantly in Thailand, the terms 'coconut sugar' and 'palm sugar' are often used interchangeably. However, coconut sugar is different both in taste, texture and manufacturing methods from palm sugar, which is made from the sap in the stems of the Palmyra palm, the date palm, the sugar date palm, sago palm or the sugar palm. Coconut trees continuously flower so harvesting of this wonderful product supports the farming families all year round.

In some villages in Sri Lanka, generations of families harvest this coconut sugar. The families looked after the coconut trees because they are their living but also because they are able to pass on their knowledge to a new generation. Coconut sugar today is processed by hand the same as it was years ago. It is essentially a two-step process. It starts with harvesting or 'tapping' the blossoms of a coconut tree. Farmers make a cut on the spadix and the sap starts to flow from the cut. The sap is then collected in bamboo containers. The sap collected is then transferred into pots and placed over moderate heat to evaporate the moisture content of the sap. The sap is translucent and is about 80 per cent water. As the water evaporates, it starts to transform into a thick syrup-like substance known as a 'toddy'. From this form, it can be further reduced to crystal, block or soft paste form. Essentially, coconut sugar's form depends on the moisture content of the toddy. Coconut sugar is subtly sweet, almost like brown sugar, but with a slight hint of caramel. However, since organic coconut sugar is not highly processed, the colour, sweetness and flavour can vary depending on different factors. Coconut sugar's colour, sweetness and flavour can vary slightly from packaging to packaging depending on the coconut species used, the season when it was harvested, where it was harvested and even the way the sap or toddy was reduced. Coconut sugar comes in crystal or granule form, block or liquid.

For the sweet-toothed, the Glycemic Index (GI) of coconut sugar is 35 and it is classified as a low GI food. By comparison, most commercial honeys are GI 55 and cane sugars are GI 68, so coconut sugar is a healthier option than refined white cane sugar and brown cane sugar. It can be used as a 1:1 sugar substitute for coffee, tea, baking and cooking. Just as the coconut itself has nutrients so does this natural product. The sap contains amino acids as well as potassium, magnesium, zinc, iron and vitamins B1, B2, B3 and B6. Unfortunately, in the production of the sugar, using moderate heat to reduce the liquid to form a solid probably destroys some of the essential nutrients, especially the B group vitamins. As well as using the flowers for coconut sugar this sap of the coconut is made into candy or sweet syrup before it is further boiled or heated to make the sugar.

Coconut Meat

The desiccated or dried coconut is commonly referred to as the 'meat'. It's worth checking the ingredients of coconut meat as lots of supermarket coconut contains a preservative called propylene glycol, to prolong its freshness or moisture content. This preservative is not necessary. Untreated coconut may be a little yellow as it has no preservative and has been naturally dried for preservation.

You can buy untreated coconut online, or try your local health food store. Once you familiarise yourself with quality brands, keep your eyes open and find more local suppliers.

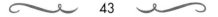

Coconut Flour

Coconut flour is packed with fibre. Plus, it adds a slight sweetness to any dish. Coconut flour is the finely ground dried coconut that is leftover after coconut oil has been extracted. Because coconut flour is very dense and absorbs liquid easily, you will need to add a little extra of the liquid ingredients when baking to keep the final result from drying out. Adding extra eggs is another way to make this product work well. When you use the product initially you may wish to substitute half the quantity with other flours until you adjust your recipe. I recommend that you store the coconut flour in the fridge or freezer as it doesn't freeze in powdered form and will be much fresher. Usually it costs much more than normal flour so you don't want it to go off before you use it all. Treats made with coconut flour are filling so are good for making you feel fuller. As there is no gluten in coconut flour it is also suitable for coeliac diets. The fibre in coconut flour is about 1¼oz (38–39g) per 3½oz (100g) of flour. It is also very high in protein, yielding about 19 grams per 100 grams. Just be aware of the potassium and sodium content for anyone on special restrictive diets.

Coconut Milk

Coconut milk is the liquid that comes from the grated meat of a coconut. It has a rich taste and colour similar to that of milk due to its naturally high fat content. Coconut milk is also a wonderful source of nutrients but make sure you read the ingredients as many of the milks and creams have added preservatives and thickeners. Canned coconut milk and cream contain guar gum. Guar gum is not well digested by many people and can cause abdominal discomfort. Once opened, cans of coconut milk must be refrigerated and are usually only good for a few days. If not refrigerated, the milk can sour and spoil easily.

Making your own milk from raw coconut

You can easily make your own coconut milk from freshly grated coconut meat.

You can make two types of coconut milk: thick or thin. Thick milk can be prepared by directly squeezing grated coconut meat through cheesecloth. To make the thinner coconut milk, take the squeezed coconut meat left in the cheesecloth and soak in warm water until cool. Then squeeze the meat a second or third time for thin coconut milk. Thick milk is mainly used to make desserts as well as rich and dry sauces. Thin milk is used for soups and general cooking.

When refrigerated and left to set, coconut cream will rise to the top and separate out from the milk.

Coconut cream

Coconut cream is taken from coconut milk, but contains less water. The difference is mainly consistency. It has a thicker, more paste-like consistency, while coconut milk is generally a liquid. Coconut cream is used as an ingredient in cooking, having a mild non-sweet taste

Coconut cream is the thick non-liquid part that separates and rises on top of the coconut milk. You can also use the Coconut Milk from powder recipe to achieve your coconut cream.

Coconut milk from powder

If you're not into that much effort but are not sure about using the

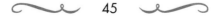

canned source, then try using quality coconut powder. Just mixing it up with water to get your desired thickness for your dish is simple and lots of traditional cooks use it.

Mix together 2 cups of water to 1 cup of coconut powder, whisking and beating, as you gradually add the water to the powder and find the consistency you need.

Creamed coconut

Creamed coconut is a coconut product produced from the meat. It is the unsweetened, dehydrated fresh meat of a mature coconut, ground to a semi-solid white creamy paste. It is sold in the form of a hard white block which can be stored at room temperature. It has an intense coconut flavour. Creamed coconut is a compressed block of coconut flesh which has been slightly dehydrated and sold in a waxy lump. In cookery, it is chopped into pieces or grated before it is added to dishes. By adding warm water it can be made into coconut milk or coconut cream. Creamed coconut is added to Indian, Thai and Asian recipes to enrich curries and sauces. In the West it is primarily used in confectionery items, ice-cream and sauces.

Coconut wine

This is an alcoholic beverage made from coconut. Coconut sap or nectar is taken from the flower clusters and used as a drink or they can be left to ferment on their own to make palm wine. With further processing by distillation the wine can be made into an alcoholic drink, known as Arrack in the Philippines. Also referred to as coconut vodka.

Heart of palm

The buds of adult coconut plants are edible and are known as 'palm cabbage' or 'the heart of the palm'. They were considered a rare delicacy as harvesting the buds of wild, single-stemmed palm trees resulted in the death of the palm tree. Through the cultivation of palm varieties that are multi-stemmed for domestic and commercial markets the heart of the palm can be found canned. Then there are the natural pests that reduce the harvest or destroy crops. So the heart of the palm are sometimes called 'millionaire's salad'.

The newly germinated coconuts contain an edible fluff of marshmallow-like consistency termed coconut sprout, produced as the endosperm nourishes the developing embryo, also considered a delicacy.

Coconut, diet and disease

The use of quality coconut products in our Western diets is quickly gaining popularity, demonstrating the coconut's versatility and practical applications in a healthy balanced diet. This nutritional product can also serve as an immune and digestive support for existing, lifelong conditions such as coeliac disease and long-term preventative and management measures in largely treatable diseases, such as adult-onset diabetes Type-2. I've included here information about the value of adding coconut to your diet in support of, but certainly not limited to, just these conditions.

Paleolithic diet movement and coconut

The paleolithic diet (abbreviated to the paleo diet movement or paleo diet), also popularly referred to as the caveman diet, Stone Age diet and hunter-gatherer diet, was made popular in the mid–1970s by Walter L. Voegtlin, a gastroenterologist.

It is fundamentally a modern nutritional plan based on the presumed ancient diet of foods that were hunted and fished during the Paleolithic era, such as meat, including offal, and seafood, eggs, insects, fruit, nuts, seeds, vegetables, mushrooms, herbs and spices that various hominid species habitually consumed during the paleolithic era—a period of about 2.5–2.6 million years which ended around 10,000 years ago with the development of agriculture and grain-based diets know as the Neolithic agricultural revolution.

Using commonly available modern foods, the 'contemporary' Paleolithic diet consists mainly of fish, grass-fed, pasture-raised meats (only lean cuts of meat, free of food additives, preferably wild game meats and grass-fed beef, since they contain higher levels of omega-3 fats compared with grain-produced domestic meats), eggs, vegetables, fruit, fungi, roots, nuts and clean filtered water and teas.

Food groups that were rarely or never consumed by humans before the Neolithic agricultural revolution are excluded from the diet, such as: grains, legumes, dairy products, potatoes, refined salt, refined sugar and processed oils and alcohol.

Some plans allow a little flexibility, like adding some processed oils from fruits and nuts, such as olive and flaxseed oil. The benefits to your health for those on a Paleo diet would be that fundamentally you are eating less refined, processed, manufactured foods with preservatives and chemical alterations and moving back to whole foods and so the philosophy is to keep things simple. By eating fresh fruit, fresh vegetables, simple grass-fed meat, nuts and oils, you would be reducing your toxic load, improving your digestive health, antioxidant intake and energy and allowing your elimination organs to do their function more effectively. People who follow and commit to making these changes to their diet I hope are also making changes to their lifestyle by exercising, because they are attempting to improve their health with the view to increasing their longevity by reducing the risk factors for the potentially diet-related preventable diseases.

On the paleo diet you would have a reduced sugar load on your pancreas supporting stable blood sugars and thus reducing the risk factor for diabetes. A cleaner and leaner dietary intake will also support and reduce your overall risk of cardiac health complications and risk of cancer. As a way of reducing obesity and weight issues, the paleo regime of nutrient-dense foods should assist a natural reduction of weight to healthy range for each individual, increasing vitality, energy and reducing the potential of developing weight-related diseases such as diabetes.

Coconut products are used as a staple fat source for those following a paleo diet. Those on the paleo diet will choose coconut oil as it fits into the dietary requirements and has lots of health benefits. It's reasonably priced, saturated, stable and has a very pleasant taste and aroma to most people. Following the paleo you can satisfy your sweet tooth with raw honey or coconut palm sugar, in small quantities.

Coeliac disease

Coeliac disease is caused by a reaction to gliadin, a gluten protein found in species of wheat, such as barley, rye, kamut and tritiacale, and subspecies spelt, semolina and durum. Some people also react to oats, although this may be simply due to cross-contamination with other grains either in the fields or during harvesting, storing and distribution of the raw product. Coeliac disease is so widespread today that there are companies that assure the 'purity' of oats and so they are still able to be consumed by coeliacs.

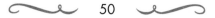

Exposure to the gluten protein found in wheat causes a reaction with the small-bowel tissue called villi. This creates an inflammatory and immune response that then leads to destruction of this lining of the small intestine (called villous atrophy). As the intestinal villi are responsible for digestion, this damage affects the absorption of vitamins and minerals from food. Most of the nutrients that are ingested in our diet are absorbed in the small intestine and transported through the walls into the bloodstream. So the villi work like very specific filters that sort and only accept the best and reject the rest. Villi also provide a protective barrier against pathogens introduced to the body via food. If someone suffering from coeliac disease continued to expose themselves to wheat, the gliadin causes damage to the villi, exposing the intestinal wall and setting off in the immune system causing antibodies to attach the body. This continuous atrophy or destruction of the small intestinal villi leads to malabsorption of vitamins and minerals, essentially leaving the person starving, not to mention the pain and discomfort this process also causes.

Coeliac disease is genetic. Sometimes the disease is triggered—or becomes active for the first time—after surgery, pregnancy, childbirth, viral infection, or severe emotional stress. Symptoms of coeliac disease vary from person to person. Symptoms may occur in the digestive system or in other parts of the body, and people with coeliac disease may have no symptoms but can still develop complications of the disease over time.

Symptoms also vary depending on a person's age and the degree of damage to the small intestine. Adults are more likely to have digestive symptoms and still be undiagnosed. Recognising coeliac disease can be difficult because some of its symptoms are similar to those of other diseases. Coeliac disease can be confused with irritable bowel syndrome, iron-deficiency anaemia caused by menstrual blood loss, inflammatory bowel disease, diverticulitis, intestinal infections and chronic fatigue syndrome. As a result, coeliac disease has long been under-diagnosed or misdiagnosed. As people and doctors become more aware of the many varied symptoms of the disease and reliable blood tests become more available, diagnosis rates are increasing.

Gluten is found mainly in foods but may also be found in everyday products such as medicines, vitamins and lip balms. Without healthy villi, a person becomes malnourished, no matter how much food they eat. The only known effective treatment is a lifelong gluten-free existence.

Coeliac and coconut

Having no gluten, coconut is a product that is a great support for those with this condition and coconut flour is an ideal substitute for wheat. It is a fine, creamy white flour that has a slight sweetness and taste of coconuts. Coconut flour as a replacement for wheat flour is an excellent provider of vital vitamins C, E, B1, B6, B3 and B5. It also contains minerals such as calcium, selenium, magnesium, phosphorous and potassium. Coconut flour can be used to make cakes, sweet breads and other desserts.

You can use coconut products in all your cooking and personal care products.

The digestive help of anti-bacterial and antiparasitic qualities and immune support with the anti-viral qualities of coconut give sufferers of coeliac disease an affordable choice of product that can enhance their health.

Coconut has essential fatty acids omega-6, which is an anti-inflammatory product and immune support. What a lovely lubricant internally and externally, helping to soothe and heal on so many levels.

By incorporating coconut into all areas of their diet can assist coeliacs to have a sustainable diet that will help give their body what it needs.

Diabetes and coconut

Coconut oil can be beneficial for people who have a family history of diabetes and reduce the risk of developing adult onset diabetes Type 2. Coconut contains medium- and short-chain fatty acids that are digested and absorbed differently to long-chain fatty acids. Our body doesn't need pancreatic digestive enzymes to break down coconut oil in the digestive tract and transport them into the bloodstream.

This means that there is less stress on the pancreas, and when combined with a low glycemic diet, you can use coconut products to maintain more stable blood sugar levels.

Today, the prevalence of diabetes means that most people know of the disease or know people with diabetes. Every cell in our bodies requires a constant source and fine balance of glucose for our metabolism, growth, repair and survival.

Type-1 diabetes is partly inherited and is also known to be triggered by certain infections. Formerly called juvenile diabetes or insulin-dependent diabetes, it is usually first diagnosed in children or teenagers. With this form of diabetes, the beta cells of the pancreas no longer make insulin because the body's immune system has attacked and destroyed them. Treatment for Type-1 diabetes includes taking insulin daily for the rest of their lives.

Type-2 diabetes is primarily caused by lifestyle factors and genetics. Known as adult-onset diabetes or noninsulin-dependent diabetes, it is the most common form of diabetes, and in many instances the most preventable.

Often people who develop Type-2 diabetes have little or no concept of the delicate balance of glucose in their system and just as often struggle constantly with understanding and managing their diet. People can develop Type-2 diabetes at any age—even during childhood. This form of diabetes usually begins with insulin resistance, a condition in which fat, muscle and liver cells do not use insulin properly. At first, the pancreas keeps up with the added demand by producing more insulin. In time, however, it loses the ability to secrete enough insulin in response to meals.

A family history of diabetes combined with being overweight and inactive all increase the chances of developing Type-2 diabetes. Type 2 can seem to be silent and latent, waiting to be triggered by these factors but it can also be triggered by stressors such as long-term physical stress or a sudden physical trauma such a major surgery, major infection or sudden grief. Treatment includes using diabetic medication, making wise food choices and being physically active for the rest of your life.

The third main form, gestational diabetes, occurs when pregnant women without a previous diagnosis of diabetes develop a high blood-glucose level. It may precede development of Type-2 diabetes in the mother.

Blood sugar regulation, pre-diabetes and hypoglycaemia

Our body works very hard every minute of the day trying to establish balance and stability to sustain life and function at a normal level. Our body requires a stable temperature and an exact amount of food.

When we put food into our mouth, our body immediately begins to breakdown molecules into smaller digestible nutrient molecules in our digestion, which is released into our bloodstream. This presence of glucose that enters the bloodstream triggers the production of insulin, a hormone that helps glucose get into cells where it can be used for energy. This process of insulin secretion lowers the level of glucose in your bloodstream and prevents it from reaching dangerously high levels. As your blood sugar level returns to normal, so does the secretion of insulin from your pancreas.

If you haven't eaten for several hours and your blood sugar level drops, another hormone from your pancreas called glucagon signals your liver to break down the stored glycogen and release glucose back into your bloodstream. This keeps your blood sugar level within a normal range until you eat again.

Once our immediate energy needs have been met, extra glucose still remaining in the bloodstream can be stored in our muscles and liver for later use in the form of glycogen.

If our muscle and liver stores of glucose are full, but we still have extra glucose floating around in our blood, then insulin can help our body store this excess sugar as fat by breaking down glycogen into smaller molecules and puts them together in the form of fat. Then the fat is transported from the liver and stored in fatty tissues in the body. Once sugar turns into fat it cannot be reversed back into glucose (sugar). The fat stays as fat until it is metabolised by the body as a fuel either in restricted diets that enable our bodies to use stored fat as energy or through exercise.

When we constantly overeat or eat incorrectly, we put extra demand on our organs and our pancreas, and the development of adult diabetes for example is a strong sign that our organs cannot cope with this overload.

The following general signs and symptoms may be indicators that your glucose mechanism is stressed and that you may need to make conscious changes to avoid the possibility of developing Type-2 diabetes in years to come.

- Constantly waking ravenous after eating the night before.
- Regular fatigue after meals
- Overwhelming fatigue and reduced mental equity between 3–5 pm in the afternoon
- Shaky and irritability before meals or if you skip meals or go without food for prolonged periods
- Migraines and headaches especially when hungry
- Mood swings—feeling down or depressed or very irritable and impatient, then feeling better from eating sugar or food of some kind
- Regular sugar cravings, at certain times of the day or particularly when stressed or tired
- Insomnia from being hungry at night, eating and then unable to get back to sleep
- Nausea when hungry from not eating a meal on a regular basis
- Most of us recognise that we suffer from some of these symptoms from time to time so make sure that you seek help to address them as they may be signs of other serious issues. But if you have a family history of diabetes, are overweight on a long-term basis and do little or no formal exercise other than your daily routine then you need to make conscious changes. Prevention is the key:
- It's your responsibility to make the changes to lead to a healthier life.
- Get help with your diet if you have no understanding of what a sensible diet is. Keep a food diary so that you are consciously aware of what goes into your mouth. Eating much smaller portions at regular intervals or every 4 hours throughout the day can assist with appetite

as well as blood sugar fluctuations.

- Gather friends or family to help you and suggest working together by initiating basic exercise, such as walking 15 to 30 minutes per day outside. Exercise improves glucose metabolism and supports insulin sensitivity.

- Drink your water, taking a sports bottle with you everywhere and increase the amount you drink over a few weeks to get to the 1½ to 2 litres daily (coconut water can be included here).

- Increase protein intake to balance complex carbohydrate and to slow assimilation of glucose into the bloodstream.

The glycemic index

The glycemic index (GI) provides a measure of how quickly blood sugar levels rise after eating a particular type of food. The effects that different foods have on blood sugar levels vary considerably. The GI estimates how much each gram of available carbohydrate in a food raises a person's blood glucose level following consumption of the food, relative to consumption of pure glucose, which has a glycemic index of 100.

Foods with carbohydrates that break down quickly during digestion and release glucose rapidly into the bloodstream tend to have a high GI; foods with carbohydrates that break down more slowly, releasing glucose more gradually into the bloodstream, tend to have a low GI. The concept was developed by Dr David J. Jenkins and colleagues in 1980–1981 as part of research to find out which foods were best for people with diabetes.

The impact a food will have on the blood sugar depends on many other factors such as ripeness, cooking time, fibre and fat content, time of day, blood insulin levels and recent activity. Use the Glycemic Index as just one of the many tools you have available to improve your dietary choices, and thus maintain better health.

- Low glycemic foods are foods than rate at 55 or less.
- Medium glycemic foods are food rated 56–69.
- High glycemic foods are foods rated 70 and above.

Your body breaks down carbohydrates from foods—such as bread, rice, pasta, vegetables, fruit and milk products—into various sugar molecules, which has an effect on your insulin levels. It is common for people who develop Type-2 diabetes later in life to have difficulty identifying or wanting to acknowledge that foods they may have enjoyed eating in the past, are converted to carbohydrates, which in turn affects their blood sugar and insulin levels.

It is our conditioning that prevents us from seeing the food that we have grown up eating as broken down into components of fats, sugars and carbohydrates. Instead, we just eat what we eat and have always eaten without really considering what it is. A dry cracker or biscuit is actually a carbohydrate, it is made from a grain, turned into flour (carbohydrate) and then a dough (carbohydrate) and cooked until crisp and is still a carbohydrate, just like a sweet biscuit but crunchy and used with savoury toppings. It still contains sugar as well as salt and converts to a carbohydrate that breaks down to a sugar and affects your insulin levels.

Carbohydrate-rich foods include:

- Starches, which are found in foods such as peas, corn, white potato
- Grains into flour—breads, sweet and dry biscuits, cakes, pastries, pasta, rice
- Legumes, split peas, lentils and dry beans such as pinto, kidney, black etc.

- Sugars, such as those naturally found in fruits and dairy products as well as packaged sweeteners and sugars added in processing.

When a person is stressed and tired or pushes past the need to sleep on a regular basis they will tend to grab high sugar and carbohydrate foods that give them a short-lived boost to their energy.

When this happens, people who are unaware that the high sugar food they just ate is the reason for their sudden drop in energy reach for another sweet or high carbohydrate food, which starts the cycle all over again. When our blood sugar is bouncing from too high to too low repeatedly throughout the day, we certainly don't feel our best. On the other hand, when our food choices help us maintain consistent normal blood sugar levels, we feel great and have the energy we need to enjoy long, active days.

However, even though fibre is considered a carbohydrate, since it is not digested (except sometimes very late in the digestive process by bacteria in the large intestine), it does not directly raise blood glucose levels.

Since most proteins and fats from food are not turned into glucose by this same process, they typically have much less of an immediate effect on our blood sugar and so by combing proteins, the right fats and low glycemic index foods we can maintain long-term health insulin–sugar balance.

Coconut sugar or coco sugar has a very low GI, making it an ideal sweetener, especially for diabetics. Coco sugar has a low GI of 35. By comparison, most commercial honeys are GI 55, and cane sugars are GI 68.

Coconut sugar is sourced from the inflorescence or flower of the coconut palm (Cocos nucifera). This flower is what eventually transforms into the coconut fruit.

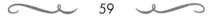

The unopened flower is thinly sliced and the sap oozing out is collected in bamboo or coconut shell containers. This sap is then boiled and concentrated to form granulated sugar.

The sugar from coconut has a nutritional content far richer than all other commercially available sweeteners. It is particularly high in magnesium, potassium, iron and zinc.

When you are a diabetic you must always take ultimate responsibility for the food you choose to eat, but coconut products can be accounted for in your diet and when used correctly, in a conscious addition to your diet, can add variety to what seems a restricted diet. So not only does coconut give you the added flavour sensation but it can also be used to boost your health and keep you on the right track. There are 30 recipes included in this book to get you started and stimulate some creativity of your own.

Coconut and immunity

Our immune system is vital to our survival. Most viruses and bacteria have a coating made up of lipids (fats) that provide them some protection from our immune system and allow them to multiply and make us very sick. Coconut oil can provide us with the means of supporting our immune system because of the medium-chain fatty acid lauric acid that is converted to monolaurin in our bodies.

As I've explained earlier in the section on oils, our bodies convert lauric acid to monolaurin that has natural anti-viral, anti-fungal and anti-bacterial properties, which means that these fats have the ability to be anti-viral, anti-fungal and anti-bacterial both internally and externally. The mechanism of action of this monolaurin works because of the MCFA being similar in structure to the virus and bacterial walls.

Viruses spread by replication and the monolaurin bind to the lipid membrane that covers the virus stopping its replication. Unable to replicate itself causes the virus to disintegrate, effectively splitting open like an over-ripe tomato.

Our immune system then sends in antibodies or white blood cells to clean the debris. If, at the initial signs of exposure to and symptoms of an illness such as the common cold, you were to have 1–2 teaspoons of coconut oil morning and night for seven days as well as quality rest and a cleaner simple diet, you may not even get the full-on symptoms and you may recover more quickly and more thoroughly. It's about priorities, rest and allow your immune system to do the job it was designed for.

Our body cleans the cells at night, so our immunity is affected and reduced if we have poor-quality sleep or fewer hours sleep than usual. In the winter, or when others around us are becoming unwell, we will be exposed to airborne germs that can lead to illness if our immune system is not supported.

People who exercise sensibly on a regular basis actively stimulate their immunity. During moderate exercise, immune cells (macrophages) circulate through the body more quickly and are better able to kill bacteria and viruses.

After exercise ends, the immune system generally returns to normal within a few hours, but consistent, regular exercise seems to keep an elevated level of immune detectors circulating and assisting your body to respond faster so you may not experience illness as severely.

To support your immune system in a more natural way, clean up your diet, get rid of the takeaway and junk food and start including whole foods, low carbohydrates and dairy for a few weeks and look at what stressors are adding to your poor immunity. Treat yourself to the coconut water Energiser Smoothie or Rejuvenation Juices in the recipe section and add some Coconut Oil on a daily basis for approximately two weeks and see what changes this brings about with your tolerance and feel the boost to your immune system.

As we all know, for changes to happen you have to make the commitment to change.

General Health

Psoriasis, eczema and mild skin infection: Clean, cold-pressed coconut oil placed on the skin can be beneficial for eczema or infections. Virgin, cold-pressed coconut oil is ideal. Fill a clean, small jar with the coconut oil and use it specifically for this purpose. By using a wooden craft stick as an applicator you can help avoid contaminating the remaining portion in the jar. Apply to the area twice per day, in the morning and evening after showering or bathing. Candida and bacterial bowel overgrowth: Taken internally, coconut oil has been known to keep the colon healthy, inhibits yeast and Candida growth and feeds the body with instant energy. For ongoing treatment of Candida I would recommend dietary measures as well as the coconut oil for three to six months of two tablespoons of oil, then followed up by a reduced dose and maintenance of dietary changes.

Enveloped viruses such as Herpes Simplex: For the treatment of enveloped viruses such as cold sores (Herpes Simplex) you can use the oil as a topical ointment on the lesion and take 1–2 tablespoons internally twice per day until the lesion is healed and then follow up with daily for

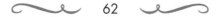

two weeks. Usually these lesions are caused by nutritional deficiency of the essential amino acid L- Lysine as well as a stressor, either emotional, immune or environmental such as extreme weather exposure (heat/ sun or bitter cold). Taken internally as suggested and up to two weeks after as a support. Follow up with looking into what is your trigger including your diet and vitamin needs.

Grazes and scratches: Grazes and scratches: Clean the wound well and, if possible, allow to air dry. Using a wooden craft stick, apply the amount of oil you wish to use to a clean finger and apply gently to the graze and cover with clean gauze. Internal dosages will also help support the immune system.

Fungal toe infections and athlete's foot: For those fungal toenails and athlete's foot, coconut oil is wonderful. Use a clean, small separate jar of oil so you can throw out what's left over at the end of treatment and use a fresh supply for the next time. Carefully clean and thoroughly dry your feet and try not to cross-infect yourself. The best way is not to use a public shower if possible. Wear open-toed shoes if you have to, and at home make sure that you scrub your shower frequently and ensure that others using your shower are not affected, causing re-infection. You may need to treat everyone to break the cycle. Remember to use one hand per foot and a separate clean towel for each foot. You can even wear latex or vinyl gloves, especially when applying the oil to the affected toes or lesions.

Simply apply the cold-compressed coconut oil from the jar using a wooden craft stick and liberally cover the infected area. Ideally this should be done twice per day until lesions are clear and then continue for a further week to ensure that the fungus or infection is not just sitting under the skin waiting to reappear. Naturally if this occurs then begin the process over. It is an affordable method with fewer toxins from pharmaceutical products and a fresh supply can be easily found if needed again. The wonderful benefit is that you will be moisturising your skin at the same time, removing any dry scaly skin from your feet. Remember to also take a tablespoon or so of the oil internally so it works as an internal and external treatment.

A healthy coconut diet

Using coconut as part of a well-balanced diet can help promote health and weight-loss. But rather than overload you with lots of diet information, I thought I would share with you the story of one of my clients and her journey with diet, making use of the wonderful coconut products available.

This lovely lady consulted me about her diet and her desire to lose weight naturally, with the view of long-term practical management. For the purpose of this book and to keep her identity private I will refer to her as Alice.

Alice is a 37-year-old mother of three. She had always struggled with her weight and always watched what she ate. She had tried many of the commercial diets and food programs over the years. Before her wedding, she went on a strict, calorie-controlled diet as lots of brides do and looked wonderful for her wedding and honeymoon. Things went along reasonably well until she had her first child. After child number one Alice found she couldn't shift the last five or so kilos. Eighteen months later, after her second child, Alice struggled with about 10 extra kilos. Being so busy with a young family, Alice didn't have the time, money or the energy to do formal exercise for herself to get into shape and just as she was gearing up for this, along came baby number three, putting her weight-loss plans on hold again. By the time Alice had come to see me she was overwhelmed by the demands in her life and her weight issues significantly affected her self-image and self-esteem.

Alice's husband, like many husbands, works long hours like many husbands and for the past two years Alice has had a part-time job. Now her youngest is at school, Alice feels that she may have more time to commit to herself and she wants to tackle her weight and lack of exercise.

Like many other working mums, Alice struggled with thinking up new and creative family meal ideas every day and had settled into a routine of easily prepared meals that everybody liked.There was a takeaway night, plus a few extra ones when things got on top of her and sometimes it might have been takeaway up to three times per week. Plus lots of other packaged food was being included, that were easy for lunches and on-the-run snacks for the children.

Because of her years of fad diets, she has an understanding of portion control, foods containing fats, carbohydrates and sugars. She was also not getting enough water, drinking not much more than 17½fl oz (500ml) of water per day above her coffee and tea intake daily.

My job as her naturopath was to help Alice with her diet and exercise, accounting for her family health as well, so Alice did not have to prepare separate food for the family. Flat out Monday to Friday, Alice really only had the weekends available to work on some preparation and planning for the rest of the week. My prescription and planning had to be practical to fit into her busy lifestyle. It also had to be simple and easy to work into her existing family diet and flexible enough to help her achieve a long-term outcome.

Initial consultation

After our initial consultation I gave Alice some homework to do before our next meeting, which was scheduled for one week later.

1. A food diary to record all her food and water intake for that week. I wanted an idea of her routine diet—the good, the bad and the ugly. I suggested this went on the fridge so it would not be forgotten to be filled in daily.

2. A food diary for Alice to put in alternative suggestions that she would like and recording times of the day where she would be able to fit in 15 minutes of walking sessions.

3. A shopping list of coconut products for her to purchase in her usual shopping places. I explained how she could gradually incorporate these products into her pantry and recipes. She could start by replacing a quarter, then a half of the products she's currently using with coconut products. This slow process of intergrating coconut products into the family diet meant that there would not be too much objection as she tried the new products. So mixing some coconut oil into her butter and frying with coconut oil instead of other oil and butter in recipes. Most children love the fragrance and taste of coconut.

4. Prescription of nutritional supplements to support Alice on a daily basis and instructions on increasing her water to 3–4 pints (1.5 to 2 litres) per day that she records in her food diary.

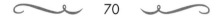

5. I wanted Alice to find one piece of clothing that she could realistically fit into in three months, something that could now fit, but was just that bit too tight and didn't feel comfortable enough to wear out, to bring along to her next consultation.

6. Alice had to make up a minimum of four new playlists on her musical device she uses to exercise with.

   • Playlist 1: 15 minutes of high-tempo songs that she loved and that she could move in a rhythm to and 5 minutes of slower cool down music

   • Playlist 2: 20 minutes of mixed-tempo music, so that if she felt tired there were songs that she could slow down and recover with and keep going to the end of her time and 5 minutes of slow, cool down music.

   • Play List 3: 25 minutes of mixed-tempo music, so that if she felt tired there were songs that she could slow down and recover to and keep going to the end of her time and 5 minutes of slow, cool down music.

   • Play List 4: 30 minutes of mixed-tempo music, so that if she felt tired there were songs that she could slow down and recover to and keep going to the end of her time and 5 minutes of slow, cool down music.

At her second consultation, I had recipes, diet and exercise routines ready for our meeting. This is where I explained to her about exchanging her usual products for coconut products, including her oil, flour and sugar and incorporating more water. I educated Alice about the benefits of coconut to increase her energy due to the medium-chain fatty acids that are easily digested and very efficiently metabolised and so important for her exercise recovery and weight loss. I also included the benefits of the lauric acid to her sugar balance and food cravings and to support her immune system. In order to be effective, Alice needed to understand how and why this simple food was so easy to incorporate into the regular favourite foods the family enjoyed. I wanted Alice motivated and excited about her new changes.

I put together a diet and exercise routine to help Alice on her journey to better health and weight loss. I have included here an average daily diet suggestion and exercise routine which can be modified depending on your own lifestyle. This diet and exercise modification for Alice was about a four-month process, with seven consultations and support sessions.

What I do is give a week of a planned menu as a suggestion and also lists of suggestions for meals and encourage clients to design their own menu. From my understanding of Alice's weekly routine this is what I suggested as a guide. Alice needed to keep a food diary and to see that she was regularly drinking water and exercising to stay motivated. Keeping this on the fridge was usually the best way to remember. I tried very hard to ensure that Alice had minimal and manageable separate meal preparation for her and her family. When on a diet plan it is not totally possible to avoid. See Appendix for charts.

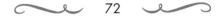

Weekly food diary and planner

For every day of the week—Monday through until Sunday—you should draw up a list of your meals.

Breakfast

Included daily in my breakfast suggestion for a week is 1 teaspoon of coconut oil to stimulate metabolism and energy each day. Medium-chain triglycerides (MCT) found in coconut oil are readily converted into fuel and used by brain cells for improved brain function. Coconut oil improves digestion and nutrient absorption, thereby supporting and promoting good general health. There is no reason why children can't have a small glass of the juice with their breakfast as well.

Psyllium husks are an important addition to your diet as they assist in appetite control by swelling up and giving you the feeling of satiety. Psyllium is a gently bulking fibre that helps to draw toxins from the bowel wall and increases bowel actions that help with waste elimination. Water intake is crucial when taking this fibre to prevent constipation and so I always encourage clients to keep the food diary and tick off the daily water consumption to ensure the 3 to 4 pints (1.5 to 2 litres) per day. Every morning before breakfast try to drink at least one glass of filtered water. Have the filtered water in a jug on the bench and in a drink bottle ready to go out the door.

Breakfast suggestions

- Hot porridge made from oats. **Hint:** Add one cup of raw oats to two cups of water in a small saucepan and sit covered overnight. In the morning just heat, boil for five minutes and serve with toppings. This saves you time in the morning and raw oats are a healthier option than commercial cereals.

- Buckwheat, rice or coconut pancakes—topped with stewed fruit, coconut milk, rice milk, almond milk, fruit juice, yoghurt and honey, LSA meal and coconut oil.
- Fresh muesli—soaked oats, chopped fruit, chia seeds, linseeds and coconut oil, topped with soymilk, almond milk, rice milk or stewed fruit, yoghurt or fruit juice.
- Wholemeal toast, rye toast, sourdough toast, multi-grain toast—topped with scrambled, poached or boiled egg, baked beans, cooked tomatoes (grilled), sardines, tuna, salmon or nut butters.
- Freshly made fruit juices from the recipe section of this book or others made with fresh fruit and vegetables in season in combinations or individually. Best consumed within 30 minutes of preparation. Delegating a job the night before to a child to wash fruit and vegetables and put into a tupperware container, ready to go in the morning will save time. Ingredients such as green apple, pear, carrot, celery, pineapple and ginger root are some good choices to get started with.
- Fresh fruit, raw nuts, yoghurt and coconut oil.
- Smoothie: banana, yoghurt (coconut milk, rice milk, almond milk), coconut oil, raw egg.
- Stir-fry: 4–5 mushrooms, 1 cup bok choy, chopped, 3½oz (100g) diced tofu, 2 eggs. Sauté mushrooms, bok choy and tofu, add and scramble eggs and serve on a slice of toast.

Breakfast menu for one week:

Monday: 7fl oz (200ml) Invigorator coconut juice (see recipe), with 1 teaspoon coconut oil and 1 teaspoon psyllium husks.

Tuesday: 1 scrambled egg and steamed and seasoned spinach on 1 slice of grained bread, drizzled with 1 teaspoon warmed coconut oil.

Wednesday: 7fl oz (200ml) detoxifier drink (see recipe) with 1 teaspoon of coconut oil and 1 teaspoon of psyllium husks.

Thursday: 2oz (60g) blueberries, 2 strawberries, 1 teaspoon warmed coconut oil mixed with 2 tablespoons plain yoghurt. Prepare the night before and add 1 teaspoon psyllium husks in the morning

Friday: 1 cup of pre-soaked oats, 6 raw pre-soaked almonds and 1 teaspoon coconut oil. Soak everything in a bowl the night before and just add 1 teaspoon psyllium husks in the morning.

Saturday: 1 lean rasher bacon, 1 poached egg, tomatoes and spinach on one slice of grained toast drizzled with 1 teaspoon of coconut oil. Vary up your weekend breakfast so you don't get bored.

Sunday: 1 coconut pancake, syrup and fruit compote. A day that feels like a treat.

Snacks

Snacks are an optional extra. They help to keep your energy up and for recovery from exercise. But remember they are just a snack not a meal. This is where Alice was encouraged to drink half her daily water by lunchtime.

Monday: 1 serve Energiser Drink (see recipe).

Tuesday: 2 protein balls and ½ serve of Energiser Drink (see recipe),

Wednesday: 2 protein balls (see recipe)

Thursday: ¼ cup berries or fruit with 1 teaspoon of psyllium husks, to provide good fibre.

Friday: 2 protein balls (see recipe)

Saturday: fresh platter of grazing finger-food and dips such as hummus

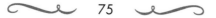

and tzatziki from the supermarket are fine for convenience—include sticks of carrot, celery, courgette (zucchini), bell pepper (capsicum), snow peas, cherry tomatoes and sprouted mung beans or alfalfa sprouts for fun.

Sunday: This is a good time for food preparation and so snacks are optional.

Lunch

For Alice, Saturday and Sunday were the best time of the week to plan meals, shop and prepare food for the week ahead. Making use of the weekend to prepare meals for those busy working days, when you are time-poor and tired, means that you will have healthy portion-controlled meals ready. If you have children, recruit the ones old enough to learn about food preparation and enlist them to help you, even if it's just to wash and prepare fruit, salad and vegetables to be made into meals and cooked.

Making some of the recipes from this book and freezing them in meal-sized portions, ready to defrost, is so much better for you than getting a takeaway. Plastic containers are fantastic for keeping cut and washed salad vegetables fresh in the fridge, ready for those quick throw-together salads for lunch and dinner.

When you are trying to eat a healthier diet, it is a good idea to make a little extra food the night before and store it in a plastic lunch container, ready for work the next day along with the rest of your daily supplies of water and snacks. When we become hungry by missing meals or not having meals prepared, it's easy to make poor food choices and eat way too much. When this happens, we sabotage our diet goals for the day, which usually results in less weight-loss and ruins your resolve to stay committed to your long-term weight-loss goals. When you know food is ready and waiting, this can curb temptation to grab something on the run, so you remain in control and on target. If you fail to plan then your plan will surely fail.

- Salad: lettuce, tomato, grated carrot, cucumber, whatever you like.
- Salad in a container with small tin of tuna, chopped chicken, ham, hard-boiled egg or homemade quiches made in muffin tins without the pastry are easily frozen and quick to grab. Handy for school lunches as well.
- Sticks of carrot, celery or cucumber and dips such as hummus or tzatziki.
- Fruit salad in a container with some raw nuts and psyllium husks.
- Dinner leftovers from the night before.
- Soups, casseroles or slow-cooked meals in winter.
- Spaghetti bolognaise and salad.
- Stir-fried vegetables.

Between lunch and dinner is the next best time to finish your daily water intake.

Lunch menu for one week:

Monday: Salad and or leftover food from Sunday dinner.

Tuesday: Laksa (see recipe) or cold hamburger and salad from the night before.

Wednesday: Extra bowl of stir-fry from the night before. Easy to make a little extra and just set aside while serving.

Thursday: Leftover shredded chicken and salad in a bowl with dressing. Just place in a container for lunch the next day, while dishing up the evening meal.

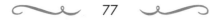

Friday: Tuna and salad with coconut and apple cider vinegar dressing.

Saturday: Garlic and Sweet Potato Wedges (see recipe).

Sunday: Fish Soup (see recipe).

Snacks

Have your fruit pre-washed on paper towel in a container in the fridge, ready for an afternoon snack. The protein balls can be kept in the fridge in portion-controlled snaplock bags for handy muchings.

Afternoon snacks for one week:

Monday: 1 thin slice of Apricot Cake (see recipe)—great for a snack and any leftovers can be frozen in portions for later use.

Tuesday: ½ cup fruit from a fruit platter of washed and sliced fruit.

Wednesday: 2 protein balls.

Thursday: ¼ cup Roasted Nuts (see recipe).

Friday: 2 protein balls.

Saturday: Rest of fruit platter.

Sunday: 4–6 pre-soaked almonds.

Dinner

Whenever you're making a meal from fresh ingredients that will freeze well, make a larger quantity and set some aside to freeze. This is a great time-saver for busy people. For example, when making spaghetti bolognaise sauce, use half for that meal and use the rest to make into a lasagne to either freeze or pop in the fridge to use in a day or two. With some crunch salad and fresh crusty bread, this is another quick time-saving healthy meal option already sorted.

Dinner menu for one week:

Monday: Homemade hamburgers (on toasted hamburger rolls) with salad and lots of dipping sauces.

Tuesday: Beef strip stir-fry and rice or vermicelli noodles.

Wednesday: Cooked chicken shredded and spread over a platter of salad vegetables.

Thursday: Chicken Nuggets (see recipe) and salad with balsamic vinegar or apple cider vinegar dressing

Friday: Spaghetti bolognaise with egg fettuccini pasta and salad.

Saturday: Fish Pie (see recipe) and salad.

½ cup chilli popcorn to snack on through the evening.

Sunday: Roast meat and lots of vegetables. Small bowl of coconut pudding for dessert.

Water

Tick off the amount of water you drink each day to help stay on target.

Portion sizes: Use a small 1½ cup bowl size for breakfast. A small 1½ cup bowl and a storage container for stir-fries and curry meals and lunch for work. And an entree plate or a bread and butter plate only for other meals.

Exercise

At our initial consultation, Alice said that she didn't have the time, money or energy for exercise.

Now that her three children were at school, I explained to her that she should consider exercise as an appointment that she would not miss. You always make sure you don't miss your hairdresser or doctor's appointment, so don't miss your exercise appointment. Book yourself in and just do it.

I suggested to Alice that she starts off doing just 15 minutes of brisk walking, three to four days per week. Weekdays needed to be fitted in around getting her children out of the house and to school. The walk was to be followed by coconut juice as a nutritional source of quick energy from the medium-chain triglycerides (MCTs) which increases energy and assist with her exercise recovery.

Exercise massages all your internal organs, stimulating your bowels and enhancing all your elimination organs, helping to eliminate waste and to manage your appetite.

Daily exercise is great for those happy hormones, which can help to relieve stress and support your immune system. Exercise stimulates neurotransmitters in your brain that then stimulate the brain's pituitary gland to release endorphins. These endorphins produce a feeling of euphoria, modulation of appetite, the release of different sex hormones and an enhancement of immune response. Cortisol is a hormone produced by the body under stress; exercise burns cortisol and can greatly assist almost everybody in our stressful lifestyle.

Regular exercise helps your cells respond to insulin and empties muscles of their stored sugar. Glycogen is stored in skeletal muscles and the liver, and regular exercise assists in using glycogen from muscles to use as energy and regulates the vital blood sugar levels, increasing insulin sensitivity that helps with appetite modulation and control. There are so many reasons why exercise is good for you and beginning with 15-minute exercise sessions is a great way to get started and increase your fitness and stamina.

Suggested walking days for Alice: Monday, Tuesday, Saturday and Sunday.

Weight and measure: At our second consultation, I weighed and measured Alice and took a photo of her in her chosen outfit. This is just a motivational tool, as you have to have small attainable goals not just a wish list. This is also a very confronting experience that requires trust and lots of encouragement. I measured Alice on week 1, week 6 and week 12. In week 12 I also took another photo so that Alice had tangible outcomes and results that supported her self-esteem and self-image. There is a chart example included in the appendix.

Self-weighing: Alice was to weigh herself on the same day and at the same time each week. After waking up, and using the toilet, she weighed herself without clothes and recorded this weight in her weekly food diary.

Water: 3–4 pints (1.5 to 2 litres) per day, managed throughout the day and finished by dinner time to enable her kidneys to flush out fluids and not disturb her vital quality of sleep with the need to go to the toilet at night.

Remember that if you fail to plan then your plan will fail.

Alice's weekly diet and exercise regime

Week 1

Exercise: Walking 15 minutes three to four times per week with her playlists for that would keep her inspired to stride. Stretching after exercise to reduce any soreness and increase flexibility. Here I instructed Alice to perform stretches at night after the children were in bed. Alice had a home yoga DVD and I suggested she use it to help her stretch each night.

Week 2

15 minutes four days per week with her music and stretches at night. This is where Alice found herself doubting her abilities to cope and felt a little unwell. We had a chat and I explained that it's not unusual to have symptoms of a detoxification of sorts, as she is stimulating toxin elimination with walking and changing aspects of her diet. Drinking the water and getting plenty of rest really helps in this stage. I suggested that she allow a 20-minute rest on the bed on the days that she isn't working to help her through this transition.

Week 3

Exercise: Increase walking 20 minutes every second day.

Week 4

Exercise: Increase walking to 20 minutes four days per week. This week was another consultation (the 3rd) for support. Alice was very excited to tell me that she had lost 6½lb (3kg), which was wonderful progress.

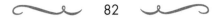

As Alice was doing her 20 minutes four days per week, I encouraged her to find a hill to include in her next week's walking. Alice did find that she was starting to walk to the songs she was listening to, without any effort, as it was an enjoyable distraction and not a chore. Alice was now managing her family diet a little better and did like the pre-freezing reminder that does make her week more organised.

Week 5

Exercise: 20 minutes four days per week with a hill included. This is a turning point as week 6 is a weigh and measure, so I really needed Alice to stay motivated to see a tangible result at our next consultation.

One of her three children had come home with a sore throat and Alice asked if the coconut oil would be O.K. for her child to take to help her immune system. I suggested that if one child has a sore throat then it is possible that the other two may suffer this over the next week. So I suggested that all three children have a week of coconut oil dosing, the two that are yet to be unwell had ½ teaspoon in the morning and the child with the sore throat was to take 1 teaspoon morning and night for one week and then ½ teaspoon for another week as a follow-up support. The children didn't object to the oil as they already liked the changes to coconut and so I suggested that she warmed the oil and gave it to them straight, with a spoonful of breakfast as a chaser. At this time I also increased some of the supplements that Alice was on as an extra support for her. With all her children likely to need extra attention it was important for Alice not to become run down herself. Alice had great compliance and three well children without sore throats, so everyone was happy.

Week 6

Exercise: 20 to 25 minutes four days per week and two hill climbs. This was Alice's fourth consultation, a day where I did her weight and measurements for some tangible results. Alice had lost 11lb (5kg) in weight and a little over 4in (10cm) overall and was really happy with herself. When someone has a good amount of weight to lose it can be less noticeable until you lose about 22lb (10kg) and begin to wear smaller clothes or more fitted clothing, showing off your new shape. This time really is about working on supporting all of the elimination organs and getting a smoother routine with water and diet and exercise leading to a healthier body.

The difference in Alice was her general attitude towards herself and her wellbeing.

Alice really enjoyed the challenge of walking and increasing the distance, using music to keep her happily distracted. This was also a very affordable means of increasing her fitness and the yoga DVD was now a good investment as she looked forward to the stretching. She'd lost a clothing size in places she didn't notice yet in her clothing.

Alice found that substituting coconut products for her usual products in her diet wasn't difficult, as the children really liked coconut. The gradual exchange of ingredients worked well to find the right balance. The texture of some of the flour products took some adjustment, and taking the coconut and psyllium in the morning was not difficult when mixing with breakfasts.

Week 7

Exercise: 20 to 25 minutes four days per week and two hill climbs.

Week 8

Exercise: 25 to 30 minutes four days per week and one hill climb.

Week 9

Exercise: 25 to 30 minutes four days per week and two hill climbs. This was Alice's fifth consultation where I ensured that Alice was getting enough nutrition and taking supplements I had prescribed, if she needed them.

Alice had lost almost 15½ lb (7 kg) happily doing her walking four times per week and two days with hills. Alice was really noticing that her jeans fitted better and she was looking through the wardrobe for other clothes that she could wear again. Alice looked much happier and even said she felt much more confident in her ability to cope and achieve her longer term weight management.

Week 10

Exercise: 25 to 30 minutes four days per week and two hill climbs.

Week 11

Exercise: 30 minutes four days per week and two hill climbs. Alice told me that she had now lost 19¾lb (9kg) ramped her 30 minutes four times per week to four hill days and was now aiming for 22lb (10kg) at our weight and measure and photo at our 12-week consultation.

Week 12

Exercise: 30 minutes 4 days per week and 2 hill climbs. This was Alice's sixth consultation and the twelfth week of her diet and exercise program. Alice was a very happy lady when she came in to see me at this consultation

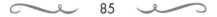

as she had lost her 22lb (10kg) as well as 15in (38cm) loss overall. She put on the outfit she had chosen in week one and wasn't at all self conscious of having her measurement taken, just a little nervous that she wasn't going to have lost much more than our last measurement. The before and after photo was a great hit and I did email her the two so that she had a record and something to keep her motivated.

From here, I suggested that Alice consider taking up some weight training or aerobic classes at her local gym. Alice was feeling really motivated and I wanted to offer her some variety to her walking and to begin to tone and strengthen her body, to maintain and continue her weight loss. In the winter this is a good alternative if the weather is just too miserable to go out.

Week 13–15

Exercise: 30 minutes three days per week and one weight-training class at her local gym.

To keep Alice motivated and to give her variety, I suggested she go the local gyms to see which one she preferred and which one had classes that would fit in with days she wanted to substitute her walk for a weight session. Alice began with a casual session payment at a gym to do one session per week. She could afford this and it was a convenient way for her work out what she liked and what worked into her regime. With her new 1½ stone (10kg) weight loss and improved shape, Alice felt confident enough to go to the gym. She said she wouldn't have considered this before due to her lack of self-confidence and poor body image.

Week 16

At week 16, Alice had her seventh consultation to consolidate her treatment. She was very happy to have continued and lost a further 6¾lb (3kg), even surviving the Christmas celebrations and family feasting that can be the undoing of a good diet schedule.

It was great to be able to help someone incorporate simple easy changes when they are ready and willing to make these changes for themselves with a little guidance. Alice was ready to explore new things and take on board my suggestions continuing to do some weight training at the gym.

Alice's total loss was 28¾lb (13kg) in 16 weeks. That's about average, allowing for the fact that Alice wasn't strictly weighing and measuring food. As Alice already knew about portion control, all she had to do was use smaller serving bowls, water, exercise and fibre to feel fuller.

When Alice was tired and hungry she had her protein balls to help her feel comforted and not gain weight like she would if she grabbed a chocolate treat or some other fast carbohydrate snack. So Alice still had her flat-out week working and managing a very busy house with three young children and still managed to make the time to walk and prepare quick, healthy meals and snacks for everybody in the house.

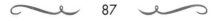

Recipes

Coconut recipes

When you start introducing a variety of coconut products into your diet, I hope you feel positive changes in your health such as increased energy, increased metabolism and better digestive health.

Coconut is healthy, adaptable, nutritious and tasty. Its versatility means that it can be incorporated into almost any dish from breakfast to dinner and snacks inbetween.

Thirty recipes are included in this book to inspire you to use coconut oil and coconut products and enjoy a healthy coconut lifestyle.

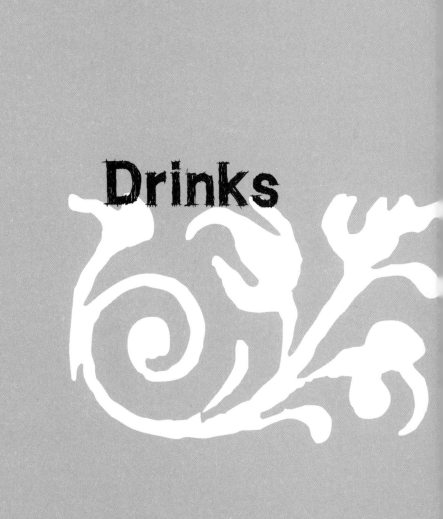

Drinks

Invigorator Juice

What a fantastic way to boost your day. This is a good liver tonic and will help stimulate metabolism.

1½ cups refrigerated coconut water (fresh is best or 1 can coconut water)

¼ cup wheatgrass juice or green powder—spirulina, wheatgrass powder, or sprouted broccoli powder, chopped parsley (whatever green food you have around)

¼ cup fresh pineapple juice

$^1/_8$ cup lime juice or lemon juice

wedge of lemon

sprig of peppermint

ice cubes

In a blender, add the coconut water, wheatgrass juice or other powder, the pineapple and lime or lemon juice and the ice cubes.

Blitz or blend to crunch up the ice cubes, pour into a tall glass, add a wedge of lemon and a sprig of peppermint. Enjoy.

Refresher

3½fl oz (100ml) coconut water
1 lime, juiced
handful of crushed iced cubes
3½fl oz (100ml) sparkling mineral water

Add coconut, lime and crushed ice cubes to a blender. Blitz and pour into a glass. Top up with sparkling mineral water.

Energiser Smoothie

A wonderful follow-up 30 minutes after your workout to replenish your electrolytes and support muscle repair and waste elimination.

1 ½ cups refrigerated coconut water (or 1 can coconut water)

¼ cup protein powder (if you are on the paelo diet or vegan, you can use rice protein rather than the whey protein from bovine sources)

1–2 tablespoons psyllium husk

¼ cup fresh berries or antioxidant powder

1 tablespoon coconut oil

ice cubes

1 capsule acidophilus powder (optional) for good digestive health

In a blender combine coconut water, protein powder, psyllium husks, berries or antioxidant, coconut oil and ice cubes and blitz until combined. If you like you can add acidophilus powder.

Consume within about 30 minutes of your workout to support your energy and post-workout recovery.

Tip: Add a heaped spoonful of coconut oil to your recovery smoothies a few times a day if you are on a mass gain program. The oil will help you stay full for longer and it will give you an energy boost that will last throughout the day. Try adding it to a fruit smoothie—you'll barely taste it once it is blended in.

Psyllium husk is found in supermarkets and health food shops. This is a wonderfully gentle fibre that supports toxin elimination and helps to support you feeling full to curb your appetite and prevent binge eating ruining your diet.

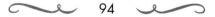

Detoxifier

1½ cups refrigerated coconut water or 1 can of coconut water

1 cup fresh blueberries, raspberries, grapes (fresh is best but frozen are OK)

a sprig of fresh peppermint leaves

juice of 1 lime or a small lemon

handful of crushed ice

Combine all the ingredients in a blender and blitz away.

Tip: Ever tried frozen grapes? Just wash and remove the stalk. Dry with a paper towel and freeze them

Snacks

This wonderful Protein Ball recipe was developed through my own need for a healthy protein snack that I could make so I could control the ingredients. After dismal taste experiences with commercial products, I made this recipe which evolved from a cooked protein cookie recipe. It was after a long busy day, and I was too tired to go to the trouble of baking so I modified the recipe and after a bit of trial and error, I think I've struck gold. I love the crunchy popping that the chia seeds add and the chocolate flavour of the protein makes me feel like I'm having a naughty treat. The psyllium husk fills me up and I know I am looking after my digestive health on many levels as well as my waist line.

For any vegan or vegetarian cooks, just use a rice protein powder made from fermented brown rice. Rice protein powder is also usually gluten-free for coeliac sufferers and fits right into the paleolithic diet.

Protein Balls

Makes approximately 30 balls

1 cup protein powder (whey or rice) with the variety of flavours pick your favourite

3 capsules acidophilus powder (optional)

¼ cup almond meal or LSA (freshly ground, if possible)

¼ cup psyllium husks

½ cup desiccated or shredded coconut

½ cup chia seeds

½ cup other nuts and seeds (linseed, activated almonds, walnuts, macadamia, sunflower, hazelnuts), roughly chopped

¼ cup coconut oil, warmed to liquid

2 tablespoons molasses or treacle (optional)

extra desiccated or shredded coconut, to roll balls

In a large bowl, combine all the dry ingredients.

Add warmed oil and molasses to bind. Add more if you need to at this stage.

Roll into teaspoon-sized balls and roll them in the extra coconut.

Store in zip-lock bags in the fridge. Four balls per bag equals 1 portion.

Note: If you're on a diet and trying to control your appetite these are fantastic. Keep them handy to curb your hunger and stay in control. Take them to work as a healthy snack option when you're peckish or at morning tea and you won't gain weight. Enjoy them guilt-free, anytime!

Chia seeds are a raw ancient seed full of omega 3 and fibre.

To make activated almonds, pre-soak raw almonds in cold water for a few hours or overnight. Drain and towel dry.

Chilli Coconut Popcorn

Makes 6 cups popped, excellent for vegan and celiac

½ cup organic popping corn

3 tablespoons virgin coconut oil, unrefined

Add to taste:

spicy chilli oil or finely chopped chilli, to taste

around ¼ tsp Celtic sea salt

drizzle of maple or agave syrup OR 2 teaspoons
    each coconut sugar and water, dissolved

Using an extra large stock pot or popcorn popping pot, add coconut oil over medium-high heat.

Drop in 2–3 kernels and cover pot with lid. Wait until first kernel pops, then add in the ½ cup popping corn. Quickly cover with lid and beware any stray popping kernels!

Shake around pan for a minute as kernels pop. Turn heat higher if needed to help along the popping—just be sure to move those kernels around so they don't burn.

After most of the corn has stopped popping, turn off the heat. Do not open lid as kernels should still be popping a bit.

Let sit until popping stops, then transfer to a large mixing bowl. Toss with spicy chilli oil, salt and desired sugar.

Serve warm.

Garlic Sweet Potato Wedges

2–4 medium sweet potatoes

2 cloves garlic, chopped

2–4 tablespoons coconut oil

2 tablespoons pepita or sunflower seeds,
coarsely chopped

1 tablespoon dried oregano

1½ tablespoons dried basil

1 teaspoon dried rosemary

Celtic salt, to taste

Preheat oven to 350°F (180°C). Wash and scrub the sweet potato, dry with paper towel and cut into wedges or chunks.

In a bowl, combine the garlic, coconut oil, seeds, oregano, basil, rosemary and Celtic salt.

Add the potato, stirring with your hands to make sure all the pieces are covered with the mixture.

Spread the wedges onto a baking tray that has been lightly greased with coconut oil.

Bake for about 45 minutes, or if you prefer them crispier, leave in oven for an extra 10 minutes.

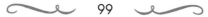

Roasted Nuts and Coconut Treat

¼ cup cold-pressed coconut oil

½ the meat of one coconut, chopped into chunks
    or slices

¼ cup raw cashews

¼ cup raw walnuts

¼ cup raw pistachios

¼ cup activated almonds

Celtic salt, to taste

In a pan, heat half of the coconut oil and cook the coconut meat until toasted. Set aside in a bowl.

Heat the remaining oil in the pan and add the nuts and toast until they begin to go crispy or turn golden. Taste one to find your desired crunch.

Add the nuts to the coconut and season with Celtic salt to taste.

Note: Activated almonds are raw, soaked almonds. What a tasty treat these are—try them in your morning breakfast yoghurt. These lovely plump, chewy sweet treats are good for your blood sugar and curbing your appetite when you are feeling peckish. To make activated almonds, pre-soak raw almonds in cold water for a few hours or overnight. Drain and towel dry.

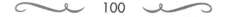

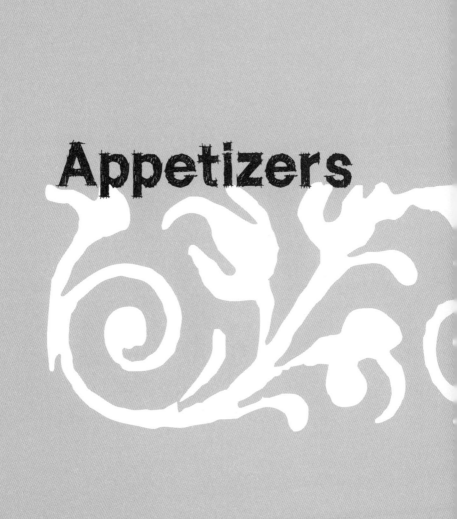

Appetizers

Thai Laksa

Serves 4

2oz (60g) vermicelli noodles

1 tablespoon coconut oil

1 clove garlic, crushed

1½ tablespoons lemongrass, finely chopped

1 teaspoon fresh ginger, finely grated

2 teaspoons red curry paste

36fl oz (1 litre) chicken stock

2 tablespoons soy sauce

1 tablespoon coconut sugar, grated

14fl oz (400ml) can coconut milk

12 medium shrimp (prawns), peeled and deveined

½ cup button mushrooms, sliced

10½oz (300g) baby spinach leaves

2 tablespoons lime juice

¼ cup cilantro (coriander), chopped

2 scallions (spring onions), thinly sliced

Soak the noodles in cold water and set aside.

Heat oil in a large saucepan over medium heat. Add the garlic, lemongrass and ginger and gently cook until fragrant. Add the curry paste and cook for 30 seconds. Add the stock, soy sauce and sugar and bring to a boil. Reduce the heat and simmer for 20 minutes.

Stir in coconut milk, shrimp, mushrooms, spinach, lime juice and cilantro. Strain soaking noodles and add to the mix. Cook for 5 minutes or until shrimp just change colour.

To serve, ladle soup and noodles into bowls. Garnish each bowl with scallions.

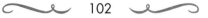

Fish Soup

1 x 14oz (400g) packet vermicelli noodles

1 stick celery, finely chopped

1 carrot, finely sliced

2 tablespoons coconut oil

9oz (250g) fresh seafood (marinara) mix or fresh white flesh fish

7oz (200g) fresh jumbo shrimp (green prawns), shelled, deveined, whole

1 tablespoon fish sauce

1 chilli, chopped to taste

2 cloves garlic, chopped

1 tablespoon Worcestershire sauce

1 x 14oz (400g) can coconut milk

salt and pepper to taste

3 small bok choy, stem and leaves chopped

Cook noodles as per instructions, drain and set aside to cool.

In a frying pan, sauté the celery and carrot in some coconut oil. Cook for about 5 minutes or until softened. Set aside.

In a large saucepan, bring 1 cup water to boil. Add the raw seafood.

Add the remaining ingredients: celery, carrot, fish sauce, chilli, garlic, Worcestershire sauce, coconut milk and season to taste. Simmer over a medium-low heat for 3–4 minutes.

Add bok choy and noodles and cook for another 1 minute.

Serve hot.

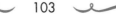

Chicken Nuggets

A fantastic healthy chicken nugget substitute for the children, made with fresh minced chicken. Double substitute and freeze half the nuggets to use as a quick hassle-free dinner with salad or dips after a busy day.

9oz (250g) minced chicken

1 egg

½ cup breadcrumbs

Celtic salt

2 cloves garlic, crushed

½in (1cm) diced lemongrass

½in (1cm) ginger, grated

1 scallion (spring onion) or chives, finely diced

¼ cup parsley, finely chopped

1 tablespoon red curry paste

4 tablespoons cold-pressed coconut oil, for frying

In a bowl, combine all the ingredients and mix well until the mixture is able to hold together. You may need to add more breadcrumbs to make this happen.

Make tablespoon-sized balls with the mixture. Set aside in the refrigerator until ready to cook and serve.

In a pan, heat the coconut oil and add the refrigerated chicken balls, in small batches so as not to overcrowd the pan. Turn and cook until golden brown and crispy. Repeat until all balls are cooked.

Toss into a gorgeous bowl and serve with the luscious Coconut Dipping Sauce (see recipe).

Tip: These chicken balls are delicious even for fussy eaters. Try them with different dipping sauces. Make double the recipe, place the nuggets on baking trays, cover with plastic wrap and freeze them. Once frozen, place the balls into a container and store in the freezer until ready to use. Simply defrost, cook and serve with salad and dip for a quick ready-meal.

Coconut Dipping Sauce

Make this sauce amd have it ready in the fridge to serve with the hot chicken nuggets when making them for adults as it may be too spicy for children.

½ cup coconut milk

2 tablespoons lemon or lime juice

2 tablespoons red curry paste

¼ cup parsley, finely chopped

¼ cup cilantrocoriander, finely chopped

Place all the ingredients in a bowl and mix until combined. Set aside in the fridge until ready to use.

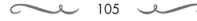

Coconut and Cucumber Nummus

The combination of coconut and cucumber is creamy, cool and soothing. Just delicious and fantastic when made from freshly caught fish.

3½oz (100g) raw, white boneless fish, sliced paper thin (refrigerate first to help you slice it)

2 cloves garlic, thinly sliced

⅓in (1cm) ginger, grated (optional)

1 red/Spanish onion, finely sliced

juice of 2–4 lemons

1 x 14oz (400g) coconut cream

1 cucumber, skinned and thinly sliced

1 bunch chives, finely chopped

salt and pepper, to taste

In a bowl, combine fish, garlic slices, ginger, onion and lemon juice to cover ingredients.

Cover and refrigerate for 30 minutes.

Strain off lemon juice. Add coconut cream, cucumber and chives and season to taste.

Chill for a further 10 minutes.

Serve.

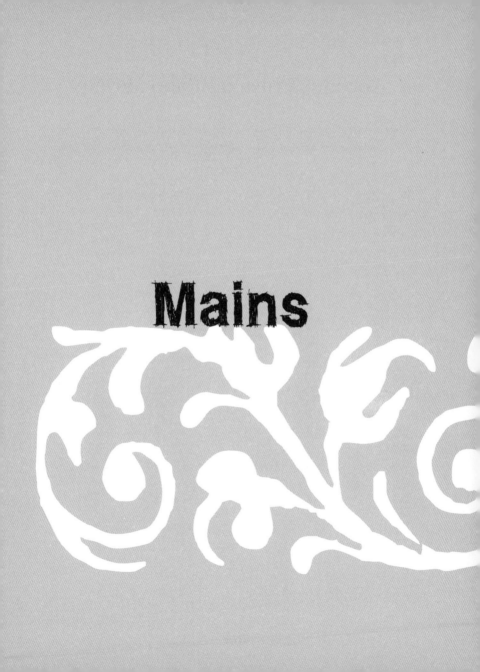

Mains

Coconut Crusted Jumbo Shrimp

Serves 4

This Coconut Crusted Jumbo Shrimp is a terrific appetiser or can be served with a bowl of rice and stir-fried vegetables as a main course.

24 large jumbo shrimp (king prawns) washed, shelled and deveined but tails left on

¼ cup dried Thai chillies

1 cup shredded coconut

½ cup all-purpose (plain) or rice flour

pinch salt

1 egg, beaten

2–3 tablespoons cold-pressed coconut oil

Peel the shrimp, leaving the tails on. Rinse and pat dry.

Grind the chillies into a fine powder in a food processor.

In a shallow bowl, mix shredded coconut, flour, salt, and 2 tablespoons of the chilli powder.

Heat the coconut oil in a large skillet.

In a bowl, whisk the egg with a little bit of water.

Dip each shrimp in the egg mixture and coat it lightly with the chilli-coconut mixture.

Fry for about two minutes on one side and another minute on the other side, or until golden brown and crispy.

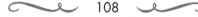

Fish Bites

Better than takeaway, you know what's inside and it's a fantastic way to introduce mild boneless fish to children. Full of protein and best eaten fresh as this doesn't freeze well.

9oz (250g) white-fleshed fish, bones removed

2–4 medium potatoes, peeled

1 egg

salt and pepper

½ cup breadcrumbs, to combine

½ to 1 cup extra breadcrumbs, to roll the patties or balls into before cooking

coconut oil, for frying

Place the fish on some aluminum foil, under a griller or broiler and cook for about 5 to 10 minutes, depending on the thickness of the fish. Separate flakes and cool fish.

Boil potatoes in a pot of salted water, until tender. Mash and cool potatoes.

In a large bowl, combine the fish and mashed potatoes. Add the egg, seasoning and breadcrumbs. Form the mixture into bite-sized balls or patties.

Roll patties or balls into the extra breadcrumbs.

Cook on a low-medium heat in coconut oil until golden on both sides.

Serve with steamed vegetables and Garlic Sweet Potato Wedges (see recipe).

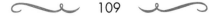

Coconut Seafood Pie

Serves 6-8, generously
We arrange a family dinner when we make this delicious fish pie.
It's always a winner. Real comfort food.

4 pearl onions, peeled and sliced

½oz (15g) butter

3 sprigs of rosemary

2 stalks celery, finely diced

1 clove garlic, crushed

1 bunch parsley, finely chopped

1 leek, diced

½ cup fish stock (either homemade or store-bought)

zest of 1 lemon

9fl oz (250ml) coconut cream

½oz (15g) all-purpose (plain) flour

5oz (150g) diced haddock or snapper

5oz (150g) firm, boneless, white-fleshed fish, diced

7oz (200g) raw shrimps (prawn), peeled

4 pieces store-bought puff pastry

Preheat the oven to 320°F (160°C).

Bring a large pot of water to the boil. Add pearl onions and simmer for 3–4 minutes

Remove onions and immediately plunge them into a bowl of ice water to stop the cooking process. Leave in water until cool, then drain and chop them. Set aside.

In a large frying pan, melt the butter over a medium heat. Add rosemary sprigs, celery, pearl onions, garlic, parsley and leek. Fry off all ingredients to bring out the aromas for 2–3 minutes or until celery softens.

Remove rosemary sprigs. Stir in the fish stock, lemon zest and coconut cream. Simmer to reduce liquid for approximately 20–30 minutes, stirring frequently.

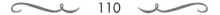

Slowly add sifted flour to thicken mixture towards end of cooking time.

In a separate frying pan, gently cook both lots of fish until flesh is white. As the fish begins to change colour, add the raw shrimp and allow all the fish to cook through with the shrimp. When all the fish has changed to white, strain off excess juice and discard. Add cooked fish and shrimp to the thickened coconut mixture. Set aside to cool.

Spray a rectangular pie dish with oil to prevent sticking. Line with puff pastry. Fill with cooled pie mixture. Seal top of mixture with puff pastry. Using a fork, prick some holes into the pastry top. Wash with egg wash to give the pie a golden brown colour.

Bake in the hot oven for 30–45 minutes or until golden brown.

Remove and serve hot.

Coconut Salmon Salad

1 tablespoon coconut oil

½ medium onion, finely chopped

2 stalks celery, thinly sliced

salt and pepper, to taste

10 ripe cherry tomatoes

7oz (200g) salmon steaks

garden salad leaves, washed and arranged on
   serving plates

1 cucumber, sliced

1 bell pepper (capsicum), sliced

1 red onion, sliced

1 bunch of Italian parsley

freshly squeezed lemon juice, to taste

Heat coconut oil in a pan. Sauté onion until opaque and add celery, salt and pepper.

Add the cherry tomatoes and move all the ingredients to one side of the pan. Add the salmon steaks and cook thoroughly, allowing the pan juices to prevent the salmon from sticking to the pan.

Meanwhile, arrange salad leaves, cucumber, bell pepper and onion on serving plates.

Transfer the salmon to the waiting salad on the serving dish and arrange tomatoes around plate.

Garnish with Italian parsley and lemon juice.

Place a liberal dollop of the gorgeous Coconut Mayonnaise onto the salmon and serve.

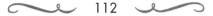

Coconut Mayonnaise

Makes about 1¹/₂ cups

1 whole egg

2 egg yolks

1 tablespoon Dijon mustard

1 tablespoon fresh lemon juice

1 pinch salt

1 pinch pepper

½ cup cold-pressed coconut oil (melted if solid)

½ cup virgin olive oil

Place the eggs, mustard, lemon juice, salt and pepper into a food processor or blender. Blend briefly for a few seconds.

With the processor or blender running on low speed, start adding your oils very slowly. Start out with drops and then work up to a thin, steady stream. This will take a few minutes.

Continue blending until all the oil is used up and blended in.

Pour into a serving bowl and use as desired.

Okra Fingers with Rice

This is a traditional Sri Lankan dish that was generously given to me to include in this book.

1 tablespoon coconut oil

17½oz (500g) okra, washed and cut into slices

1 onion, finely chopped

2 sprigs curry leaves, remove the individual leaves and remove the leaves at the end of cooking if desired

2 teaspoons curry powder

3 cloves garlic, crushed

pinch saffron powder

salt, to taste

1 tablespoon dried fish (Maldives dried fish), chopped or 1 tablespoon fish oil or fish paste

1 piece goraka (Garsinia flower) available in any Sri Lankan shop (optional if unavailable)

¼ cup coconut milk

1 cup coconut rice per person

Preheat the oven to 350°F (180°C).

Heat a tablespoon of coconut oil in a frying pan over a medium-high heat. Fry the okra slices for 2 minutes to soften and to remove prickles on the outside of the vegetable. Set aside the fried okra in an ovenproof dish.

In a bowl, combine the onion, curry leaves and powder, garlic, saffron, salt, dried Maldive fish and goraka.

In a large frying pan, heat 1 tablespoon coconut oil and gently fry the onion mixture for a few minutes to enhance the spices.

Add coconut milk and bring to the boil. Immediately take off the heat.

Pour the coconut milk mixture over the fried okra. Bake slowly in the oven until okra is tender. Serve with coconut rice.

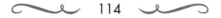

Coconut Rice

7fl oz (200ml) coconut cream

7fl oz (200ml) water

9oz (250g) basmati rice

1 teaspoon Celtic salt

Mix the coconut cream and water in a pot. Add the basmati rice and the salt.

Bring to the boil. Reduce the heat and simmer for 10–12 minutes.

Drain and serve.

This is a smooth and creamy rice. A lovely fragrant complement to your dishes.

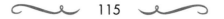

Beef Curry with Eggplant

serves 4

Beef

2 tablespoons coconut oil

14oz (400g) braising beef, such as osso bucco
   or other quality beef you like, cut into chunks

3 cups coconut milk

4 kaffir lime leaves

1¾fl oz (50ml) soy sauce

5oz (150g) coconut sugar, grated

Eggplant

1 large eggplant, cut into ¾in (2cm) thick rounds

1¾fl oz (50ml) soy sauce

3½oz (100g) cornflour starch

10½fl oz (300ml) coconut oil

Curry

9fl oz (250ml) coconut cream

4 tablespoons curry paste

14fl oz (400ml) reserved beef cooking liquid,
   set aside

3½fl oz (100ml) fish sauce

3½oz (100g) coconut sugar, grated

1 stick lemongrass, finely chopped

4 kaffir lime leaves

2–3 red chillies, chopped, to taste

1 bunch fresh basil leaves (Thai is good for this
   dish), chopped

1 bunch cilantro (coriander) leaves, to garnish

1 cup coconut rice per person

Beef

Preheat the oven to 320°F (160°C).

In a frying pan, heat the oil over a medium-high heat and brown off all the meat.

Transfer this to a casserole dish and add the coconut milk, lime leaves, soy and sugar. Cover and cook in the oven for 2½ hours or until the meat is tender.

When cooked, remove the meat and set aside.

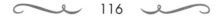

Keep about 14fl oz (400ml) of the cooking liquid aside also.

Eggplant

While the meat is cooking, combine the eggplant slices and soy sauce in a large bowl and set aside for about 30 minutes then drain.

Coat the eggplant in the cornflour.

Heat the oil in a frying pan until hot and fry the eggplant slices until golden and crispy.

Remove and drain on paper towel.

Curry

Heat the coconut cream in a large saucepan until the cream begins to separate. Add the curry paste and cook for 3 minutes

Add the reserved cooking liquid and the fish sauce, sugar, lemongrass and lime leaves

Bring to a boil and add the beef until heated through.

Add the eggplant, red chillies, basil and stir gently until combined and heated through.

Serve with hot coconut rice.

Garnish with extra coriander leaves.

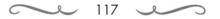

Sri Lankan Lamb

36oz (1kg) lean leg of lamb

2–4 tablespoons coconut oil

1 onion, finely diced

2 cloves garlic, crushed

2 cloves

½ cinnamon stick

1 teaspoon cardamom powder

2 teaspoons curry powder

2 pandan leaves (available from Asian
    supermarkets)

3 curry leaves

2½cm (1in) fresh ginger, chopped

1 cup coconut milk

1 tablespoon roasted curry powder (black)

Cook the lamb on a roasting tray in the oven at 350°F (180°C) for one hour or until cooked.

Cool and cut into cubes and then thin slices.

In a large frying pan, heat 2 tablespoons of coconut oil over a medium-high heat. Brown off all the meat and set aside.

In the same pan, heat 2 tablespoons of coconut oil and gently cook the onion, garlic, cloves, cinnamon stick, cardamom powder, curry powder, pandan and curry leaves and ginger for 1–2 minutes to bring out the flavour. Add the meat into the pan and cook until the meat is coated with the mixture.

Add the coconut milk and 1 tablespoon of roasted curry powder (black).

Simmer for 4–5 minutes. Remove from the heat and take out the curry leaves and pandan leaves and discard.

Serve with rice.

Filipino Shrimp Supreme

Given to me by a gorgeous lady who added the pumpkin to sweeten it up, making it more appealing to her children. To make it an adult dish just add more chilli to spice it up.

2 tablespoons coconut oil

2 cloves garlic, chopped

1 tablespoon fresh ginger, chopped or grated

1 red chilli, chopped (or more if you want it spicy!)

1 cup pumpkin, cut into about 1in (2cm) cubes

1 teaspoon salted shrimp paste

1 x 14fl oz (400ml) coconut cream

36oz (1kg) fresh, washed, shelled and deveined shrimp (prawns)

In a frying pan, heat the coconut oil over a medium heat and cook the garlic, ginger and chilli until aromatic.

Add the cubed pumpkin and fry for about 5–10 minutes or until all the pumpkin is tender.

Remove half the pumpkin and set this aside to include at the end.

Add the salted shrimp paste and the coconut cream to the pumpkin still in the pan.

Using a masher, mash the pumpkin in the pan until smooth.

Add the shrimp and cook for 3–4 minutes or until they change colour to pink.

Add the remaining pumpkin that was set aside and heat through.

Serve with coconut rice.

Vegetable Korma Curry

Serves 4

4 tablespoons cold-pressed coconut oil

1 large onion, finely chopped

2 cloves garlic, finely chopped

¾in (2cm) ginger, finely chopped

3 cardamom pods, split

2 tablespoons curry paste

1 tablespoon tomato puree

2 x 14oz (400g) can chopped tomatoes or 28oz (800g) fresh tomatoes, chopped

1 teaspoon ground coriander

1 teaspoon cumin

1 teaspoon turmeric

Celtic salt and ground pepper, to taste

17½oz (500g) seasonal vegetables, chopped into small bite-sized pieces

3½oz (100g) red lentils

17½fl oz (500ml) chicken or vegetable stock

7fl oz (200ml) coconut milk

coconut rice and fresh cilantro (coriander), to serve

Heat 2 tablespoons of coconut oil in a large saucepan.

Fry the onion, garlic, ginger and cardamom for 2 minutes. Add the curry paste, tomato puree and chopped tomatoes. Cook for a further 3 minutes.

In a separate frying pan, heat the remaining 2 tablespoons of coconut oil.

Add the spices and cook off for 1 minute to bring out the aroma.

Add the chopped vegetables and lentils and cook for 5 minutes.

Take off the heat and transfer the vegetables and lentil mixture to the pot with the tomato mixture

Add the stock and the coconut milk and bring to a simmer.

Simmer, stirring frequently until the vegetables are tender. Serve with hot coconut rice and garnish with coriander.

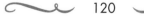

Vietnamese Chicken Curry

serves 4

2 tablespoons cold-pressed coconut oil

14oz (400g) chicken breast, diced

7fl oz (200ml) chicken stock

2 stalks lemongrass

2–3 red chillies, to taste

4 cloves garlic, chopped

¾in (2cm) ginger, grated

1 tablespoon curry powder

10½fl oz (300ml) coconut milk

4 tablespoons coconut sugar

2½fl oz (75ml) fish sauce

10 cherry tomatoes

½ medium red onion, chopped

1 handful cilantro (coriander) leaves, chopped

1 handful Thai basil leaves, chopped

Heat 2 tablespoons of the oil in a large frying pan and fry off the chicken until crispy and golden.

Add the chicken stock and bring to the boil. Reduce the heat and simmer for 20 minutes. Remove the chicken pieces and place onto a plate. Set the stock aside.

In the same frying pan, heat 2 tablespoons of oil and cook off the lemongrass, chillies, garlic, ginger and curry powder until fragrant.

Put the spice mixture into a blender and whiz to a smooth paste.

Add 3½fl oz (100ml) of the reserved chicken stock, the spice mixture, coconut milk, sugar and fish sauce and bring to the boil.

Reduce the heat to a simmer again and add the tomatoes, onion, coriander, basil and the chicken that was set aside.

Warm through and serve on its own or with coconut rice.

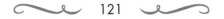

Lamb Curry with Nuts and Coconut Milk

1¾oz (50g) cashews

2 cloves garlic, chopped

½ teaspoon chilli powder

½oz (15g) fresh ginger

½ teaspoon ground coriander

½ teaspoon turmeric powder

1 bunch cilantro (coriander), chopped

½ teaspoon pepper

2–3 tablespoons coconut oil

1 small onion, chopped

36oz (1kg) lamb, diced

1 x 14fl oz (400fl oz) coconut milk

¼ teaspoon saffron

1¾oz (50g) almonds, slivered

Celtic salt

6 curry leaves (available from Asian shops)

Grind, pound or blend or blitz the cashew nuts, garlic, chilli powder, ginger, ground coriander, turmeric, coriander leaves and pepper.

Heat 2 tablespoons of coconut oil in a pan, add the onion and fry until golden, then add the blended spices and fry for a further 5 minutes to activate the aromas of the herbs.

Gradually add the meat and and fry for 5 minutes, then pour on the coconut milk. Add the saffron, almonds and salt and cook, covered, over low heat for about 1 hour, until the meat is tender and the sauce has thickened.

Sprinkle on the curry leaves.

Serve with coconut rice, of course.

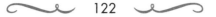

Toasted Coconut and Lime Shrimp

¼ cup sweet coconut flakes

1 tablespoon coconut oil

36oz (1kg) jumbo shrimp (large prawns), shelled, deveined and butterflied

½ tablespoon scallions (spring onions), finely chopped

½ tablespoon garlic, minced

¼ cup lime juice

¼ cup rice wine vinegar

½ cup sake or dry white wine

1 cup coconut cream

1 teaspoon vanilla extract

1 tablespoon sesame oil

salt and pepper, to taste

lime slices and/or green onion flowers for garnish

In a non-stick frying pan, toast coconut flakes over a low-medium heat until light golden brown. Remove and set aside.

Heat the coconut oil in a frying pan over medium heat. When the oil is hot enough, carefully add the shrimp and cook them for about two minutes. Quickly remove the prawns from the pan and set aside.

Add the scallions to the frying pan. Cook until opaque, then add the garlic and the acidic liquids (lime juice, vinegar and wine).

Reduce the mixture by half and add the coconut cream and stir in.

Add the shrimp, chopped scallion, vanilla, and sesame oil and cook the prawns all the way through.

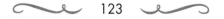

Desserts

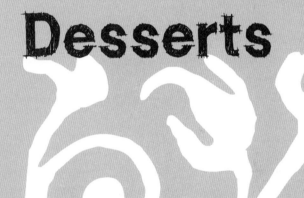

Coconut Ice-Cream

makes about 500ml
Use your ice-cream maker and follow the instructions from there.

3 egg yolks (yolks alone will give even more
    richness)

1¾oz (50g) coconut sugar or superfine (caster)
    sugar

9fl oz (250ml) coconut milk

3½fl oz (100ml) full cream milk

2 fresh vanilla beans, scraped and seeds
    removed or 4 tablespoons real vanilla extract

4 tablespoons coconut sugar, grated

Possible flavouring options:

½ cup your favourite berries, chopped or
    blended to a puree

¼ cup fresh mint, finely chopped

¼ cup mixed nuts, chopped

zest of lemon, lime or orange

3 tablespoons raw honey

¼ cup dark chocolate chips or flakes

Combine egg yolks and sugar in a stainless steel bowl.

In a saucepan, add the coconut milk, full cream milk, vanilla bean seeds and
the rest of the sugar and bring to a boil.

Immediately remove from the heat and allow to cool for about 5 minutes

Pour milk mixture slowly into the egg yolk mixture, whisking constantly.

It is crucial to constantly whisk at this point to prevent the eggs from cooking.

Once combined, strain the mixture through a sieve and refrigerate until cold.

Add your own flavours or a combination of whatever you like.

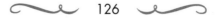

Coconut Toffee

This goes exceedingly well with coconut ice cream.

9oz (250g) coconut sugar, grated
3½fl oz (100ml) water

Combine the sugar and water in a small pot and warm until sugar has dissolved.

Now bring to the boil and immediately reduce to a constant bubbling simmer.

Continue to simmer gently until mixture is thick and sticky and a toffee consistency.

Line a flat baking tray with baking paper. To make toffee shards, drizzle the toffee all over the tray in fine threads using all the toffee mixture.

Allow to sit at room temperature and when you're ready to serve your ice-cream just break the toffee threads into pieces and use as a garnish on the ice-cream.

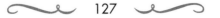

Pancakes

The consistency of these pancakes are different from ones made with wheat flour and takes some adjusting to. The recipe works best if you blend 1 cup of coconut flour and 1 cup of another type of flour such as rice, wheat, buckwheat or other until you find the mix that suits your taste.

1 cup coconut flour, sifted

1 cup rice flour or wheat flour, sifted

1 teaspoon baking powder

2 tablespoons coconut sugar, grated

pinch salt

4 eggs, separated

1 cup coconut milk

¾oz (25g) warmed, melted coconut oil

coconut oil, for frying

bananas, sliced

blueberry, raspberry or strawberry compote

goat's cheese fromage

In a medium-sized bowl, sift the flours and baking powder together. Stir in the sugar and salt.

In another bowl, beat in egg yolks, milk and oil together and then fold them into dry ingredients and whisk the mixture together to fluff it up.

In another bowl, beat the egg whites with a pinch of salt until soft peaks form, then, using a metal spoon, fold this into batter mixture.

In a non-stick frying pan, heat up some coconut oil and add two tablespoons of pancake batter into the pan.

Cook for 1–2 minutes and flip when bubbles start appearing on the surface. Cook the other side for a further 1–2 minutes.

Have a warmed plate in the oven and transfer cooked pancakes to warmed plate and keep covered until all batter is used.

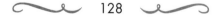

Layer pancakes with sliced banana and coconut sugar syrup and top with Coconut Ice Cream or Coconut Sugar Syrup (see recipes).

Spread goat's cheese onto pancakes and top with gorgeous compote of your choosing.

Tip: An easy compote is about 9oz (250g) of your choice of fruit, washed and hulled if needed, placed in a small saucepan.

Grate ½ cup of coconut sugar into the saucepan and bring to a gentle simmer. As sugar dissolves and fruit cooks down you get a quick and easy, a scrumptious treat for your pancakes.

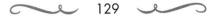

Coconut Sugar Syrup

This gorgeous syrup is really easy to make, has low GI and rivals commercial syrups in taste.

17½oz (500g) coconut sugar, grated

1 vanilla bean, scraped and seeds removed

10½fl oz (300ml) water

In a saucepan, combine the coconut sugar, vanilla and water.

Bring to a boil then reduce to a simmer for 10 to 15 minutes or until desired syrup thickness. Set aside for pancakes.

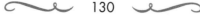

Chocolate Cake

7oz (200g) coconut oil, warmed and melted

7oz (200g) block 85% chocolate bar, melted

12 eggs

½ cup coconut milk

2 tablespoons stevia powder

1 cup coconut sugar, grated

1 teaspoon Celtic salt

2 vanilla pods, scraped and seeds removed

1 cup coconut flour, sifted

1 teaspoon baking powder

Preheat the oven to 350°F (180°C). Line and grease a 8in (20cm) round cake tin. In a bowl, combine the melted coconut oil and chocolate together and allow to cool slightly.

In a large bowl, beat the 12 eggs. Add the coconut milk, stevia, coconut sugar, salt and vanilla.

In a medium-sized bowl, sift the coconut flour and baking powder together.

Gradually mix the cooled oil and chocolate mixture into the egg mixture, making sure that it has cooled enough not to cook the eggs as you combine the two ingredients.

Now whisk the flour mixture into the batter until there are no lumps.

Pour into the greased cake tin and bake for about 40 minutes. Check if a skewer comes out clean. If not, leave to cook for 7-minute intervals and check until cooked and skewer comes out clean.

Alternately, pour into cupcake moulds and bake at 350°F (180°C) for 15 to 20 minutes, again checking with a skewer if they are fully cooked.

Cool. Decorate with icing and enjoy.

Apricot Coconut Cake

I love the combination of coconut and apricots. With all the seeds and low GI ingredients, it's just the trick for weight loss.

½ cup walnuts

½ cup sunflower seeds

1 cup coconut sugar, grated

1 cup coconut flour, sifted

1 cup rice flour, sifted

1 cup chia seeds

2 cups dried apricots, finely chopped

½ cup shredded coconut

½ cup coconut oil

2 cups coconut milk

6 eggs, beaten

Preheat the oven to 350°F (180°C). Line a tin (12 x 4in/30 x 10cm) with baking paper.

In a blender, blitz the walnuts and sunflower seeds into smaller pieces.

In a bowl, mix together the dry ingredients. Gradually add the oil, milk and then the eggs and mix together until you get a cake batter. Add more coconut milk if the consistency is too thick.

Pour into the lined baking tin and cook for 50 minutes. If a skewer inserted into the middle of the cake comes out clean, it is cooked.

Cool on a cake rack until cold. Once cold, frost with Lemon Frosting (see recipe).

Tip: Make this cake in a muffin tin or a loaf tin and freeze in portions for handy snack or lunchbox treats for school.

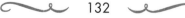

Lemon Frosting

This frosting with coconut is just divine on the Apricot Coconut Cake.

1oz (30g) coconut oil

3½oz (100g) cream cheese

1 teaspoon lemon rind, finely grated

1½ cups confectioners' (icing) sugar, sifted

shredded or desiccated coconut, to decorate

Beat the coconut oil, cream cheese and lemon rind in a bowl until light and fluffy.

Gradually add sifted sugar and mix until all combined.

Spread on the cold cake and sprinkle shredded or desiccated coconut on top to decorate.

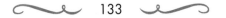

Coconut and Quinoa Pudding

½ cup coconut meat

1 teaspoon coconut oil

1 cup quinoa grain, rinsed and drained

2 x 14fl oz (400ml) cans coconut milk

1 cup coconut sugar

fresh fruit of your choice such as blueberries,
     bananas or mangoes, washed and sliced

Cut the fresh coconut meat into slices. Using a non-stick pan, add 1 teaspoon of coconut oil. Heat the oil and gently toast the coconut slices until they turn golden and crunchy.

Place the quinoa in a large saucepan with the coconut milk and coconut sugar.

Bring to the boil and then reduce and simmer, covered, for 20–25 minutes until thick and creamy.

When the quinoa is soft and cooked, layer the pudding mix with your desired fruit, in individual bowls

Top each bowl with toasted coconut for decoration and indulge.

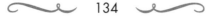

Watalapan—Sri Lankan Pudding

17½oz (500g) coconut sugar, grated, also known as palm sugar

3 cups thick coconut milk

10 eggs

2 vanilla beans, split and seeds scraped

2 teaspoons ground nutmeg

3½oz (100g) raw cashews, chopped

This pudding cooks steam so find a bowl that sits in a deep pot that can be easily removed.

Add grated coconut sugar and coconut milk in a bowl.

Continuously stir until palm sugar dissolves.

Strain liquid and set aside into the bowl used to steam.

In a separate bowl, whisk together the 10 eggs.

Pour into coconut mixture. Add vanilla and nutmeg.

Sprinkle cashews over the top and cover with plastic wrap to steam.

In a large saucepan, bring about ¾in (2cm) of water to boil.

Put bowl with mixture into the pot with the water to steam.

Put lid on the saucepan and gently simmer for 45 minutes.

Remove from the heat and the pot and allow to cool.

When cold, the pudding is set firmly enough to cut into cubes.

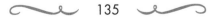

Acknowledgements

Without the support of my wonderful husband Peter who suffered (only as a man can) constantly with the introduction of new foods and diet trends ,all to the eventual benefit of his health. He is a true alpha male and a true hunter-gather and thankfully has now (eventually) embodied my passion for a healthy lifestyle. When I told him I was writing this book has proffered his own fish soup recipe with coconut milk then his fish pie as well.

My beautiful daughter Rebecca—because of the diversity of her health issues when she was young, she became my major reason for obtaining my degree. She is now a healthy adult.

To my gorgeous son—he accepts his own good health and healthy eating and does so with grace.

For my parents, who are sadly no longer with me. A special thanks to my father who passed away from a treatable illness, which inspired me to help others, to ensure no-one else loses someone they love for no reason.

Thanks to my clients who present me with challenges in health that have benefited from my years of continued studies and helping to refining my methodology in attaining a healthier existence for all—where would I be without you all?

Thanks to Linda Williams for asking if I would like the challenge of writing a book.

Last, but by no means least, thank you to my major supplier: Mother Nature in all her glory.

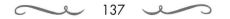

Appendix

Weekly Food Diary and Planner

Week —	Monday	Tuesday	Wednesday	Thursday	Friday	Saturday	Sunday
BREAKFAST Every morning before breakfast try to drink at least one glass of filtered water. Have the filtered water in a bottle ready to go out the door.							
SNACK Snacks are optional extra. Great to keep your energy up and for recovery from exercise. This is when you should try to drink half your daily water by lunch time.							
LUNCH Between lunch and dinner is the next best time to finish daily water so that you're not waking at night to go to the toilet.							
SNACK This snack time would be with the children after school.							
DINNER							
WATER Ticking off your water intake each day helps to stay on target.	****						
EXERCISE: Type & duration							
WEIGHT:							

Weight and Measurement Chart:

Measurements	Week 1	Week 6	Week 12	Total of loss
Bust: Nipple line				
Chest: Under breast				
Natural Waist				
Belly – Largest part				
Hips – Top of thigh/groin				
Thighs – Largest part	R: L:	R: L:	R: L:	R: L:
Arms – ½ way from shoulder to elbow	R: L:	R: L:	R: L:	R: L::
Total				
Weight:				

References

Bijlsma. Nicole.2012. *Helathy Home, Healthy family*.Joshua Books. QLD. Australia

Oseicki H. 1998. *The Physician's Handbook of Clinical Nutrition.* BioConcepts. QLD. Australia.

Davies s; Stewart.A. *Nutritional Medicine*.1987. Pan Books. London.

Murray M; Pizzorno J. 1998. *Encyclopaedia of Natural Medicine.* 2nd Edition. Little, Brown and Company. England.

Bioconcepts. 1998. *Orthoplex Technical Manual.* 6th Edition. Bioconcepts. QLD. Australia.

McCance M; Huether SE. 1994. *Pathophysiology—Biolological Basis for Disease in Adults and Children.* Mosby-Year Book Inc. Missouri. U.S.A.

Fife.Bruce.2004. *The Coconut Oil Miracle.* Piccadilly Books.

Sébédio, J. L. and Christie W.W. 2009. *Metabolism of trans-fatty acid isomers. In: Trans Fatty Acids in Human Nutrition* (2nd edition), Oily Press, Bridgwater.

Cabot. S. 1997. *The Liver Cleansing Die*t. Australian Print Group. VIC. Australia.

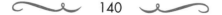

First published in 2013 by
New Holland Publishers
London • Cape Town • Sydney• Auckland
www.newhollandpublishers.com

Garfield House 86–88 Edgware Road London W2 2EA United Kingdom
Wembley Square First Floor Solan Road Gardens Cape Town 8001 South Africa
1/66 Gibbes Street Chatswood NSW 2067 Australia
218 Lake Road Northcote Auckland New Zealand

A catalogue record of this book is available at the British Library and at the
National Library of Australia

ISBN: 9781742574271

10 9 8 7 6 5 4 3 2 1

Managing Director: Fiona Schultz
Publisher: Linda Williams
Project editor: Jodi De Vantier
Designer: Tracy Loughlin
Production director: Olga Dementiev
Printer: Toppan Leefung Printing Limited

Follow New Holland Publishers on
Facebook: www.facebook.com/NewHollandPublishers